OSTEOPOROSIS

DIET MEAL PREP

COOKBOOK

Delicious and Nutrient-Rich Recipes to Prevent and Treat Osteoporosis Naturally

Melissa Daniel

Copyright© 2024 by Melissa Daniel

All rights reserved worldwide.

Warning-Disclaimer

Table of Contents

The osteoporosis diet cookbook greets you by leading you through a culinary path designed to increase bone density and improve general health. Osteoporosis, a condition associated with weakened bones and increased chances of fractures, affects millions of people worldwide. However, diet plays an essential role in keeping our bones healthy, and this book aims to show people how diverse and delicious food can be while still being beneficial to the bones.

This cookbook will introduce you to recipes rich in vital nutrients for good bone health, such as calcium and vitamin D, magnesium, potassium, and vitamins K and C. As well as having great nutritional value, these meals have flavors that can be prepared according to different dietary requirements.

Let us explore how nutrition affects bone health, starting with the basics of osteoporosis. With this knowledge base about nutrition to keep our bones healthy, we can make informed choices on what we eat. The recipes in this book, however, go beyond just strengthening your bones; they also contribute towards maintaining good health of your heart since they focus primarily on whole grains, lean proteins, and a plethora of fruits and vegetables that one might prefer eating. These dishes cater to every type of taste bud, whether it's a single person cooking, family, or friends coming over.

Every recipe has easy instructions, and nutritional information is below each. We've got you covered, from comforting soups like stews to vibrant salads, substantial entrées, or even mouthwatering desserts- ensuring your meals remain exciting and balanced.

Remember that this is no ordinary recipe collection but rather a tool for change in lifestyle habits. It is not just about what one eats but also about enjoying what one eats in order to lead better lives by developing solid bones instead of weak ones. Let's delve into this yummy journey together with one recipe at a time; hence, I welcome you all into my Osteoporosis Diet Cookbook, where health and flavor marry perfectly on your plate.

What is osteoporosis?

Osteoporosis is characterized by weakened bones, resulting in decreased density and thickness. Individuals with osteoporosis have a significantly higher risk of experiencing fractures. Usually, bones are dense and robust enough to support body weight and withstand various impacts. However, with age, bones naturally lose some density and self-regeneration capacity. In osteoporosis, bones become excessively fragile and weak, significantly increasing fracture susceptibility.

Types of osteoporosis

Primary Osteoporosis:

1. Postmenopausal Osteoporosis: The type is prevalent in women after menopause. The decrease of estrogen during menopause causes an increased rate of bone resorption, which results in weakened bones. Women have lower peak bone mass as well as hormonal changes that take place during menopause, and therefore, they become more vulnerable to this condition than men.

2. Senile Osteoporosis: Type II osteoporosis usually happens in males and females aged 70 years and above. As a person grows old, the ability of the body to produce new bone tissue declines gradually, leading to loss of bone mass over time. Trabecular (spongy) and cortical (hard) bones are affected by this type.

Secondary Osteoporosis:

This type results from certain medical conditions or treatments that interfere with bone health. It can affect both men and women at any age.

Causes of osteoporosis

Osteoporosis results from imbalances in bone resorption (bone breakdown) and bone formation. Aging often brings about a situation where the rate of bone resorption overcomes that of bone formation, leading to a reduction in bone density and strength. Osteoporosis can be developed as a result of several factors:

1. Age: The highest point of bone density is realized at an early adult age, after which it starts to decline with aging. As you age, the possibility of contracting osteoporosis increases, with women being especially at high risk after menopause.

2. Hormonal Imbalances: After menopause in women, estrogen levels reduce dramatically, leading to a fast decrease in bone mass. In addition, testosterone production declines gradually among males as they age, affecting bone mass.

3. Genetic Factors: A family history of osteoporosis, mainly if a parent had a history of fractures, can increase the risk.

4. Nutritional Factors: Both are crucial for bone health. Low calcium diets and inadequate amounts of vitamin D (which helps your body absorb calcium) contribute to decreased mineralization of bones, premature skeletal aging, and higher risks for fractures. Among them are conditions like anorexia or bulimia or having a consistently nutrient-deficient diet that weakens bones.

5. Lifestyle Choices: Lack of exercise will cause weak bones. Proper weight-bearing exercises will ensure good bone health. High alcohol intake disrupts growth and replacement in bones, usually by promoting poor nutrition, rendering the process impossible.

6. Certain Medications: Some drugs, such as long-term corticosteroids and certain antiepileptic medications, may lead to low BMD.

7. Medical Conditions and Treatments: Disorders such as Crohn's disease or celiac disease where absorption is affected; hyperthyroidism or hyperparathyroidism, which affects hormonal balance; cancer treatments, including chemotherapy as well as radiotherapy were known to lead to osteoporosis too.

Symptoms of osteoporosis

Osteoporosis, often referred to as a "silent disease," is one that can progress over many years without showing any signs until a fracture occurs. Nonetheless, some signs and symptoms may indicate its presence or risk:

1. Minimal Trauma Fractures: The most important and noticeable symptom of osteoporosis is a fracture from little injury or, in severe cases, just actions such as bending down or coughing. Commonly involved sites are the hip, spine, and wrist.

2. Back Pain: This pain can be both intense and chronic from fractured or collapsed vertebrae.

3. Loss of Height with Time: In people with osteoporosis, the spine may compress, gradually decreasing height due to fractured or collapsed vertebrae.

4. Stooped Posture or Kyphosis: This stooping posture may be brought about by vertebral fractures and weakening of spinal bones hence being commonly referred to as a "dowager's hump."

5. Bone Pain or Tenderness: Few people may experience generalized bone pain throughout the body.

Health Benefits of an Osteoporosis Diet for Women

A diet for osteoporosis that involves a lot of specific nutrients can benefit women, especially in halting or slowing the onset of osteoporosis. Women develop osteoporosis more frequently because of hormonal changes, particularly after menopause. Here are some key benefits of an osteoporosis-friendly diet for women:

1. Increased Bone Density: For constructing and maintaining strong bones, you must include lots of calcium and vitamin D in your meals. Calcium accounts for most minerals found in bones, while vitamin D is necessary for calcium absorption.

2. Reduced Risk of Fractures: Osteoporosis diets can significantly reduce the risk of fractures by improving bone density and strength, which are very common and risky among aged women.

3. Hormonal Balance: A well-balanced diet containing phytoestrogens (such as soy products) can help maintain hormonal balance, which is especially essential following menopause.

4. Improved Overall Nutrition: The diet also encourages various nutrient-dense foods such as fruits, vegetables, lean proteins, and whole grains that benefit overall health.

5. Weight Management: Weight management has been proven possible with an equally balanced osteoporotic meal alongside regular exercises. Maintaining a healthy weight is essential, as obesity puts one at risk for fractures.

6. Reduced Inflammation: Omega-3 fatty acids present in fish have anti-inflammatory properties that may assist in reducing bone loss, among others, in an osteoporotic dining plan.

7. Muscle Strength: Good protein intake should be observed for muscle health. Muscles help improve balance, thus reducing chances of falls, resulting in low incidence rates of fractures.

8. Prevention of Other Diseases: Not only does this type or kind or brand or sort or style or model or version etcetera of diet benefit bones, but it also aids in heart health; hence, it could prevent other diseases like diabetes and some cancers.

Foods to eat for Osteoporosis Diet

Focusing on specific nutrients that promote bone health is essential for an osteoporosis-friendly diet. Here are key food groups and examples that should be included:

1. Calcium-Rich Foods:

- ✓ Dairy Products: (Milk, yogurt, cheese)
- ✓ Leafy Green Vegetables: (Kale, collard greens, broccoli, and bok choy)
- ✓ Fortified Foods: (Some cereals, plant-based milk alternatives, and orange juice)
- ✓ Fish with Bones: (Canned sardines and salmon)
- ✓ Green Leafy Vegetables: (Spinach, kale, Swiss chard, and turnip greens.)
- ✓ Other Vegetables: (Brussels sprouts, broccoli, and cabbage.)

2. Vitamin D Sources:

- ✓ Fatty Fish: (Salmon, mackerel, and tuna)
- ✓ Egg Yolks.
- ✓ Fortified Foods: (Many dairy products, cereals, and some types of orange juice)
- ✓ Sunlight: (Moderate sun exposure can also help the body produce vitamin D)

3. Magnesium-Rich Foods:

- ✓ Nuts and Seeds: (Almonds, pumpkin seeds, chia seeds, and flaxseeds.)
- ✓ Whole Grains: (Brown rice, oatmeal, whole wheat.)
- ✓ Legumes: (Black beans, chickpeas, and lentils.)

4. Potassium-Rich Foods:

- ✓ Fruits: (Bananas, oranges, apricots.)
- ✓ Vegetables: (Sweet potatoes, potatoes, tomatoes, and spinach.)

5. Foods High in Omega-3 Fatty Acids:

- ✓ Fatty Fish: (Salmon, mackerel, and sardines)
- ✓ Plant-based Sources: (Flaxseeds, chia seeds, walnuts)

6. Protein:

- ✓ Lean Meats: (Chicken, turkey, lean cuts of beef and pork.)
- ✓ Plant-based Proteins: (Beans, lentils, tofu, tempeh, and edamame.)
- ✓ Meat, shellfish.
- ✓ Seeds: (Pumpkin seeds, squash seeds.)

Foods to Avoid for Osteoporosis Diet

When managing osteoporosis, certain foods and substances can have a detrimental effect on bone health and should be limited or avoided:

1. **High-Salt Foods**
2. **Caffeine**
3. **Soft Drinks, Especially Colas**
4. **Alcohol**
5. **High-Oxalate Foods**
6. **Red and Processed Meats**
7. **Wheat Bran**
8. **Excessive Vitamin A**
9. **Trans Fats**
10. **Certain Gluten-Containing Foods**

Berry Blast Protein Smoothie

Preparation Time: 5 minutes Cooking Time: 0 minutes Serving: 1-2

Ingredients

- 1 cup of mixed berries
- 1 banana
- ½ cup of Greek yogurt
- 1 scoop protein powder
- 1 cup of almond milk
- 1 tbsp chia seeds or flaxseeds
- A handful of spinach or kale (optional)
- Honey or maple syrup (optional)
- Ice cubes (optional)

Instructions

1. Combine the mixed berries and bananas in a blender. In the case of frozen fruit, add ice cubes.
2. Add Greek yogurt, almond milk, protein powder, chia seeds, or flaxseeds. Alternatively, you can also include optional kale or spinach for additional nutrients.
3. Blend until smooth on high speed. If necessary, add more milk to attain the desired thickness.
4. Extra sweetness may be obtained by tasting it with honey or maple syrup if needed. You may mix it one more time shortly.
5. For optimal flavor and texture, serve the smoothie in glasses immediately after pouring.

Nutritional (per serving)

Calories: 350 kcal Protein: 25 g Calcium: 30% (DV) Vitamin D: Varies Fiber: 7 g

Green Goddess Protein Smoothie

Preparation Time: 5 minutes Cooking Time: 0 minutes Serving: 1-2

Ingredients

- 1 cup of fresh spinach leaves
- 1 ripe banana
- ½ avocado
- 1 scoop protein powder
- 1 cup of unsweetened almond milk
- 1 tbsp chia seeds or flaxseeds
- ½ cup of Greek yogurt
- A few mint leaves
- 1 tbsp honey or maple syrup (optional)
- Ice cubes (optional)

Instructions

1. Blend the spinach leaves, banana, and avocado in a blender.
2. Incorporate one scoop of protein powder and chia seeds or flaxseeds.
3. Put almond milk and Greek yogurt into the blender.
4. If desired, throw mint leaves into the blender accompanied by sweeteners like honey or maple syrup.
5. Press blend on high speed until smooth and creamy. If it is too thick, add more milk for desired consistency
6. Serve immediately in glasses for a perfect taste.

Nutrition (per serving):

Calories: 300 kcal Protein: 25 g Calcium: 30% Vitamin K: High Fiber: 8 g Healthy Fats: High

Tropical Paradise Protein Smoothie

Preparation Time: 10 minutes Cooking Time: 0 minutes Servings: 1

Ingredients

- 1 cup of fresh spinach
- 1/2 cup of Greek yogurt
- 1/2 cup of canned pineapple chunks in juice
- 1/2 banana
- 1/4 cup of orange juice
- 1 tbsp chia seeds
- 1 scoop vanilla whey protein powder (or plant-based protein powder)
- Ice cubes (as needed)

Instructions

1. Blend spinach, Greek yogurt, pineapple chunks, banana, orange juice, chia seeds, and protein powder in a blender.
2. Blend until smooth after adding a few ice cubes. If necessary, increase the consistency with more orange juice or water.
3. Taste for sweetness and add honey or agave syrup as desired.
4. Serve immediately.

Nutrition (per serving):

Calories: 350 kcal Protein: 25g Calcium: 30% of daily value Vitamin D: Varied

Almond and Chia Seed Pudding

Preparation Time: 10 minutes Cooking Time: 0 minutes Servings: 2

Ingredients

- 1/4 cup of chia seeds
- 1 cup of almond milk (unsweetened)
- 2 tbsp honey or maple syrup (adjust to taste)
- 1/2 tsp vanilla extract
- A pinch of salt
- Optional toppings: Sliced almonds, fresh berries, or a sprinkle of cinnamon

Instructions

1. Combine the chia seeds, almond milk, honey (or maple syrup), vanilla extract, and a pinch of salt in a bowl. Then, stir thoroughly until well mixed.
2. Cover tightly with the bowl's lid and keep in the fridge for 4 hours or more overnight, which is better. The chia seeds absorb the liquid and enlarge, giving it a pudding-like consistency.
3. Once set, please give it a good stir. Alternatively, add more almond milk to make it thin if it is too thick.
4. Serve in bowls or glasses and sprinkle with sliced almonds, fresh berries, or cinnamon to taste and richer nutrition content.

Nutrition (per serving):

Calories: 200 kcal Protein: 6g Calcium: 25% of daily value Magnesium: 30% of daily value Fiber: 10g

Spinach and Feta Omelette Roll

Preparation Time: 15 minutes Cooking Time: 10 minutes Servings: 2

Ingredients

- 4 large eggs
- 1/4 cup of milk
- Salt and pepper, to taste
- 1 tbsp olive oil
- 2 cups of fresh spinach, chopped
- 1/2 cup of feta cheese, crumbled
- Optional: Fresh herbs (such as dill or parsley), finely chopped

Instructions

1. Whisk eggs, milk, salt, and black pepper in a bowl until you have a uniform mixture.
2. Place the olive oil in a non-stick pan and warm it up over medium heat. Add spinach and cook for 2-3 minutes until it collapses.
3. Pour the egg mixture into the spinach. Allow to cook without stirring until the bottom is set but the top remains liquid; this should take around five minutes.
4. Sprinkle feta cheese crumbs on one half of the omelet. Let cook for another 1-2 minutes.
5. Carefully fold the omelet in half by taking one side over the filling, then gently roll over to the other side as though making a roll. Leave it covered for another minute so that the rolls can harden.
6. At last, take your omelet roll from the skillet to a plate and cut it into two equal halves using a knife while garnishing with fresh herbs if required.

Nutrition (per serving):

Calories: 300 kcal Protein: 20g Calcium: 25% of (DV) Iron: 15% of (DV)

Quinoa Breakfast Bowl

Preparation Time: 10 minutes Cooking Time: 20 minutes Servings: 2

Ingredients

- 1/2 cup of uncooked quinoa
- 1 cup of water or milk
- 1/2 tsp cinnamon
- 1 apple, diced
- 1/4 cup of walnuts, chopped
- 2 tbsp raisins or dried cranberries
- Honey or maple syrup, to taste
- Optional toppings: Sliced bananas, fresh berries, a dollop of Greek yogurt, or a sprinkle of chia seeds

Instructions

1. Wash quinoa with cold water. Add water (or milk) to quinoa in a pan. Boil it, then reduce the heat and simmer for 15-20 minutes or until the quinoa is dry and absorbs liquid.
2. Mix in cinnamon, diced apple, walnuts, and raisins. Cook an extra 2-3 minutes.
3. Take off from the heat. Sweeten with honey or maple syrup if desired. Serve warm.
4. Garnish with sliced bananas, fresh berries, Greek yogurt, or chia seeds for extra nutrients and taste.

Nutrition (per serving)

Calories: 350 kcal Protein: 8g Fiber: 6g Calcium: 5% of daily value

Yogurt Parfait with Nuts and Berries

Preparation Time: 10 minutes Cooking Time: 0 minutes Servings: 2

Ingredients

- 2 cups of Greek yogurt
- 1/2 cup of granola
- 1/2 cup of mixed berries
- 1/4 cup of nuts
- Honey or maple syrup, to taste
- Optional: A sprinkle of chia seeds or flaxseeds for extra omega-3s and fiber

Instructions

1. Place one spoonful of Greek yogurt at the bottom of the two glasses or bowls.
2. Cover the yogurt with granola.
3. Cover with a layer of mixed berries and top with a dusting of almonds.
4. Pour another layer of berries and almonds to finish, and keep layering until the glasses or bowls are complete.
5. You can pour more honey or maple syrup on top if you want more sweetness.
6. The parfaits can be chilled for up to an hour before serving, but serving them right away will yield the most excellent texture.

Nutrition (per serving)

Calories: 400 kcal Protein: 20g Calcium: 20% Magnesium: 15% Fiber: 5g

Salmon and Avocado Toast

Preparation Time: 15 minutes Cooking Time: 0 minutes Servings: 2

Ingredients

- 2 slices of whole-grain bread
- 1 ripe avocado
- 4 oz smoked salmon
- 1 tbsp lemon juice
- Salt and pepper, to taste
- Optional: Red onion slices, capers, fresh dill, or a sprinkle of sesame seeds

Instructions

1. Toast the whole-grain slices of bread according to what amount of crispness you prefer.
2. Mash the avocado with lemon juice, salt, and pepper in a bowl. Choose to make it chunky or smooth according to your preference.
3. Spread mashed avocado on each piece evenly.
4. Place the smoked (or cooked) salmon on top of the level of avocado.
5. Add toppings such as red onion slices, capers, and fresh dill, or sprinkle sesame seeds for more taste and texture if desired.
6. Serve immediately while they are still fresh and crunchy.

Nutrition (per serving):

Calories: 350 kcal Protein: 20g Fiber: 5g

Cottage Cheese and Pineapple Bowl

Preparation Time: 10 minutes Cooking Time: 0 minutes Servings: 2

Ingredients

- 1 cup of cottage chees
- 1 cup of fresh pineapple, diced
- 1 tbsp honey or maple syrup (optional)
- Optional toppings: Chopped nuts, coconut flakes, a sprinkle of cinnamon or chia seeds

Instructions

1. First, cut the ripe pineapple into small sizes
2. Divide the curds into two equal parts using bowls.
3. On top of the curd, put the small pieces of pineapple
4. If you want sweetness, pour honey or maple syrup.
5. To make it sweeter and healthier, sprinkle your nuts, coconut flakes, cinnamon, or chia seeds.
6. Eat them when they are still fresh.

Nutrition (per serving):

Calories: 200 kcal Protein: 14g Calcium: 20% Vitamin C: High Fiber: 2g

Sweet Potato and Turkey Hash

Preparation Time: 15 minutes Cooking Time: 20 minutes Servings: 2

Ingredients

- 1 large sweet potato, peeled and diced
- 1/2 lb ground turkey
- 1 bell pepper, diced
- 1 small onion, diced
- 2 cloves garlic, minced
- 2 tbsp olive oil
- Salt and pepper, to taste
- Optional: Fresh herbs (like parsley or thyme), red pepper flakes, or a sprinkle of paprika

Instructions

1. Heat 1 tbsp of olive oil over medium heat in a large skillet. Cook sweet potato dice until soft but still slightly hard to the bite for about 8-10 minutes. Remove from skillet and set aside.
2. In the same skillet, add ground turkey. While it's cooking, break it into smaller pieces as you go along until it browns and is no longer pink. Salt and pepper it.
3. Put bell pepper dice, onion dice, and minced garlic on top of the turkey in a skillet. Cook till tender (about 5-7 minutes).
4. Sweet potato that has been cooked should be returned to the skillet. Stir so that the ingredients mix well.
5. For extra taste, one can use optional herbs or even red pepper flakes or paprika if need be. Taste with salt and pepper as necessary and serve warm as hash.

Nutrition (per serving):

Calories: 400 kcal Protein: 25g Vitamins: Vitamin A Fiber: 5g

Cherry Almond Overnight Oats

Preparation Time: 10 minutes Cooking Time: 0 minutes Servings: 2

Ingredients

- 1 cup of rolled oats
- 1 cup of almond milk
- 1/2 cup of cherries
- 2 tbsp almonds (sliced or chopped)
- 2 tbsp chia seeds
- 2 tbsp honey or maple syrup
- 1/2 tsp almond extract (optional)
- A pinch of salt

Instructions

1. Put oats, cherries, almonds, and chia into a bowl or a jar and add honey, salt, and almond extract to the mixture.
2. Cover with a lid or wrap the top of the jar tightly with plastic wrap to avoid air getting in.
3. In the morning, give your oats a good stir. If they are too thick, adjust their consistency by adding more milk.
4. If you want to, serve it topped with extra almonds and cherries.

Nutrition (per serving):

Calories: 400 kcal Protein: 10g Calcium: 20% Magnesium: 20% Fiber: 11g

Mushroom and Spinach Egg Scramble

Preparation Time: 10 minutes Cooking Time: 10 minutes Servings: 2

Ingredients

- 4 large eggs
- 1 cup of fresh spinach, chopped
- 1 cup of mushrooms, sliced
- 1/4 cup of milk
- 1 tbsp olive oil or butter
- Salt and pepper, to taste
- Optional: Grated cheese, herbs, and a pinch of garlic powder

Instructions

1. Whisk eggs, salt, milk, and pepper in a bowl.
2. Olive oil or butter should be heated on medium heat in the skillet. Add mushrooms to it once it is soft and browned (about five minutes).
3. It will take between 1 and 2 minutes for the spinach you have added to the same skillet to wilt.
4. You can pour this mixture into the skillet with mushrooms and spinach leaves. Let it stay for some seconds without stirring, then scramble the eggs gently to taste.
5. If preferred, use grated cheese and herbs. Mix them.
6. Serve egg scramble hot; feel free to add more salt and pepper according to your preference.

Nutrition (per serving):

Calories: 300 kcal Protein: 20g Calcium: 15%

Berry Chia Pudding

Preparation Time: 10 minutes Cooking Time: 0 minutes Servings: 2

Ingredients

- 1/4 cup of chia seeds
- 1 cup of almond milk
- 1 tbsp honey or maple syrup
- 1/2 tsp vanilla extract
- 1 cup of mixed berries
- Optional toppings: Additional berries, a sprinkle of granola, or a dollop of Greek yogurt

Instructions

1. In the bowl, mix the almond milk and chia seeds. Make sure that all chia seeds have been thoroughly mixed.
2. Mix in honey (or maple syrup) and vanilla extract again.
3. Wrap up the container and keep it in a fridge for overnight, or at least six hours. The liquid will be soaked by chia seeds, thus increasing their size and resulting in a pudding-like consistency.
4. Fresh berries, if used, wash them as required, then chop. Should you use frozen berries, let them thaw overnight in your refrigerator.
5. After setting the chia pudding, stir it once more. Lastly, layer glasses or bowls with berries alternating with the chia pudding.
6. If preferred, sprinkle some more granola with extra fruits or a dollop of Greek yogurt.

Nutrition (per serving)

Calories: 250 kcal Protein: 6g Omega-3 Fatty Acids: High Calcium: 25% Fiber: 10g

Spinach and Mushroom Omelette

Preparation Time: 10 minutes Cooking Time: 10 minutes Servings: 1

Ingredients

- 2 large eggs
- 1 cup of fresh spinach, chopped
- 1/2 cup of mushrooms, sliced
- 1 tbsp olive oil or butter
- Salt and pepper, to taste
- Optional: Shredded cheese (such as cheddar or Swiss), diced onions, or herbs

Instructions

1. Mix the eggs thoroughly with a bowl pinch of salt and pepper.
2. Heat half the butter or olive oil over medium heat in a nonstick skillet. Once the mushrooms are tender and have taken on some color, add them and simmer. Take out and place aside from the skillet.
3. Add the spinach to the same skillet and heat until it wilts. Take it out of the skillet and place it aside alongside the mushrooms.
4. To the skillet, add the remaining butter or oil. Pour them in and tilt the skillet to ensure equitable distribution of the whisked eggs. Cook until the tops of the eggs are still a little runny, but the bottoms are set.
5. Arrange the spinach and sautéed mushrooms on one half of the omelet. If using, add cheese, onions, and seasonings.
6. Over the filling, fold the remaining half of the omelet. Cook for a further minute or until the cheese (if using) melts. Serve immediately.

Nutrition (per serving)

Calories: 300 kcal Protein: 20g Vitamins: High in Vitamin A and D Iron: Good source

Greek Yogurt Parfait

Preparation Time: 10 minutes Cooking Time: 0 minutes Servings: 2

Ingredients

- 2 cups of Greek yogurt
- 1/2 cup of granola
- 1/2 cup of mixed berries
- 2 tbsp honey or maple syrup
- Optional toppings: A sprinkle of chia seeds, sliced almonds, or shredded coconut

Instructions

1. Start by layering Greek yogurt in the bottom of the two glasses or bowls.
2. Cover the yogurt with a layer of granola.
3. Sprinkle a layer of mixed berries on top.
4. Continue layering until the glasses or bowls are complete, and then top with a layer of berries.
5. If you would like more sweetness, drizzle with honey or maple syrup.
6. Add extra garnishes like shredded coconut, sliced almonds, or chia seeds if desired.

Nutrition (per serving):

Calories: 350 kcal Protein: 20g Calcium: 20% Fiber: 4g

Avocado Toast with Smoked Salmon

Preparation Time: 15 minutes Cooking Time: 0 minutes Servings: 2

Ingredients

- 2 slices of whole-grain bread
- 1 ripe avocado
- 4 oz smoked salmon
- 1 tbsp lemon juice
- Salt and pepper, to taste
- Optional toppings: Red onion slices, capers, fresh dill, a sprinkle of sesame seeds, or a drizzle of olive oil

Instructions

1. Toast the whole-grain bread until the texture is as crisp as you like.
2. Mash the avocado with salt, pepper, and lemon juice in a bowl. You can make it smooth or leave it lumpy, depending on your desire.
3. Over the toasty bread slices, equally distribute the mashed avocado.
4. Place a layer of smoked salmon over the avocado.
5. Optional garnishes include sesame seeds, fresh dill, red onion slices, capers, and a sprinkle of olive oil.
6. Enjoy the avocado toast immediately while it's fresh and flavorful.

Nutrition (per serving):

Calories: 350 kcal Protein: 20g Fiber: 7g Vitamin D: Good source

Overnight Oats with Almond Butter

Preparation Time: 10 minutes Cooking Time: 0 minutes Servings: 2

Ingredients

- 1 cup of rolled oats
- 1 cup of almond milk (or any milk of your choice)
- 2 tbsp almond butter
- 1 tbsp chia seeds
- 1-2 tbsp honey or maple syrup (adjust to taste)
- 1/2 tsp vanilla extract
- A pinch of salt
- Optional toppings: Sliced bananas, berries, a sprinkle of cinnamon, or extra almond butter

Instructions

1. Mix the rolled oats, almond milk, chia seeds, almond butter, maple syrup or honey, vanilla, and a pinch of salt in a bowl or jar.
2. Stir everything together until well combined.
3. Cover it and put it in the refrigerator for at least six hours.
4. Stir the oats up well in the morning. If you feel the mixture is too thick, add more milk to suit your desired thickness.
5. Put sliced bananas and berries on top of your cereal, sprinkle with cinnamon or pour some almond butter.

Nutrition (per serving):

Calories: 350 kcal Protein: 12g Fiber: 9g Calcium: 25%

<u>Veggie Breakfast Burrito</u>

Preparation Time: 15 minutes Cooking Time: 10 minutes Servings: 2

Ingredients

- 2 large whole-grain tortillas
- 4 large eggs
- 1 cup of spinach, chopped
- 1/2 cup of bell peppers, diced
- 1/2 cup of mushrooms, sliced
- 1/4 cup of onions, diced
- 1/2 cup of black beans, rinsed and drained
- 1/4 cup of shredded cheese (such as cheddar or pepper jack, optional)
- 1 tbsp olive oil
- Salt and pepper, to taste
- Optional toppings: Salsa, avocado slices, or Greek yogurt

Instructions

1. Warm olive oil in a frying pan over medium heat. Add onions, bell peppers, and mushrooms. Saute until the vegetables become tender for about five minutes.
2. Into the skillet, add spinach and black beans. Cook till the spinach wilts, approximately two minutes.
3. In a dish, mix eggs with salt and pepper. Pour into vegetable-coated pan. Cook without stirring until firmly set.
4. You can warm tortillas in the microwave or use a skillet for that purpose instead.
5. Place egg and vegetable mixture on tortilla wraps evenly. Split them; otherwise, if you want, sprinkle some cheese on top.
6. Bring both sides of each tortilla towards the center to cover its content inside.
7. Serve hot burritos with optional salsa, avocado, or Greek yogurt dollop on the side.

Nutrition (per serving):

Calories: 450 kcal Protein: 25g Fiber: 8g Vitamins: High in Vitamins A and C

Blueberry Oatmeal Pancakes

Preparation Time: 15 minutes Cooking Time: 10 minutes Servings: 2

Ingredients

- 1 cup of rolled oats
- 1/2 cup of whole wheat flour (or all-purpose flour)
- 1 tbsp baking powder
- 1/2 tsp cinnamon
- 1 cup of milk (or almond milk)
- 1 large egg
- 2 tbsp honey or maple syrup
- 1 tsp vanilla extract
- 1 cup of fresh blueberries
- Cooking spray or butter (for the pan)

Instructions

1. In a blender, pulse the oats until powdery and flour-like.
2. Mix the ground oats, flour, baking powder, and cinnamon in a bowl.
3. Mix milk with egg-whisked honey or maple syrup in another bowl. Combine this mixture with a dry one and stir to obtain uniformity.
4. Fold the blueberries gently in.
5. Grease a non-stick skillet or griddle and heat it over medium fire. Pour 1/4 of the batter for each pancake. Cook until there are bubbles on top, then turn it over, cooking till all sides turn golden brown,
6. If desired, serve them hot with extra blueberries, honey maple syrup, or yogurt.

Nutrition (per serving)

Calories: 350 kcal Protein: 12g Fiber: 6g Calcium: 20%

Almond and Banana Smoothie

Preparation Time: 5 minutes Cooking Time: 0 minutes Servings: 2

Ingredients

- 2 ripe bananas
- 2 tbsp almond butter
- 1 cup of almond milk
- 1/2 cup of Greek yogurt
- 1 tbsp honey or maple syrup
- A pinch of cinnamon
- Ice cubes (optional for a colder smoothie)

Instructions

1. Blend the bananas, Greek yogurt, almond milk, honey (or maple syrup), almond butter, and a dash of cinnamon in a blender. If you want your smoothie colder, add some ice cubes.
2. Process the mixture at high speed until it becomes creamy and smooth. To get the right consistency, you can add a little extra almond milk if the smoothie is too thick.
3. If needed, taste the smoothie and adjust the sweetness. If necessary, increase the amount of honey or maple syrup.
4. For optimal flavor, pour the smoothie into glasses and serve right away.

Nutrition (per serving)

Calories: 300 kcal Protein: 10g Healthy Fats: High Calcium: 25%

<u>Veggie and Feta Frittata</u>

Preparation Time: 15 minutes Cooking Time: 20 minutes Servings: 4

Ingredients

- 6 large eggs
- 1/4 cup of milk
- 1/2 cup of feta cheese, crumbled
- 1 cup of spinach, chopped
- 1 bell pepper, diced
- 1 small onion, diced
- 1 cup of cherry tomatoes, halved
- 1 zucchini, sliced
- 2 tbsp olive oil
- Salt and pepper, to taste
- Optional: Herbs such as basil or parsley for garnish

Instructions

1. Preheat your oven to 375°F (190°C).
2. Mix the eggs, milk, pepper, and salt in a bowl.
3. Heat the olive oil in a skillet that is oven-safe to medium. Add the bell pepper, zucchini, and onion. After around five minutes, sauté until softened. Cook the spinach until it wilts by adding the cherry tomatoes and spinach.
4. Scatter the feta cheese crumbles on top of the veggies.
5. Cover the cheese and veggies with the egg mixture. Allow it to simmer for two to three minutes, stirring occasionally, or until the edges firm.
6. Place the skillet inside the oven. Bake the frittata for 15 to 20 minutes or until it is firm and has a hint of color.
7. Let the frittata cool for a few minutes. Garnish with fresh herbs, slice, and serve.

Nutrition (per serving)

Calories: 300 kcal Protein: 18g Calcium: High Vitamins: High in Vitamins A and C Iron: Good source

Whole Grain Cereal with Nuts and Berries

Preparation Time: 5 minutes Cooking Time: 0 minutes Servings: 2

Ingredients

- 1 cup of whole-grain cereal
- 1 cup of milk or almond milk
- 1/2 cup of mixed berries
- 1/4 cup of mixed nuts
- Optional: A sprinkle of chia seeds or flaxseeds for extra omega-3s and fiber

Instructions

1. Separate the cereal made of whole grains into two bowls.
2. Over the cereal in each bowl, drizzle milk or almond milk.
3. Top the cereal with a mixture of chopped nuts and berries.
4. You can optionally add flaxseeds or chia seeds on top for added nutrition.
5. To enjoy the best texture and freshness, eat right away.

Nutrition (per serving):

Calories: 350 kcal Protein: 10g Fiber: 7g Calcium: 30%

Coconut Yogurt with Tropical Fruit

Preparation Time: 10 minutes Cooking Time: 0 minutes Servings: 2

Ingredients

- 2 cups of coconut yogurt
- 1/2 cup of fresh pineapple, diced
- 1/2 cup of mango, diced
- 1/2 cup of kiwi, sliced
- 2 tbsp shredded coconut (unsweetened)
- Optional: A drizzle of honey or agave syrup for added sweetness, a sprinkle of chia seeds or chopped nuts for extra texture and nutrients

Instructions

1. Slice the kiwi and chop the mango and pineapple.
2. Arrange the diced pineapple, mango, and kiwi slices in two dishes or glasses among the coconut yogurt.
3. Every serving should have shredded coconut on top. You can add a sprinkling of chia seeds or chopped almonds for extra nourishment, or you can drizzle with honey or agave syrup.
4. Enjoy this tropical yogurt parfait immediately for the freshest taste.

Nutrition (per serving):

Calories: 300 kcal Protein: 6g Calcium: 30% Vitamin C: High Fiber: 4g

Buckwheat Pancakes with Berries

Preparation Time: 15 minutes Cooking Time: 15 minutes Servings: 4

Ingredients

- 1 cup of buckwheat flour
- 1 tbsp sugar (optional)
- 1 tsp baking powder
- 1/2 tsp baking soda
- 1/4 tsp salt
- 1 egg
- 1 1/4 cups of buttermilk (or milk of choice)
- 2 tbsp unsalted butter, melted
- 1 cup of mixed berries
- Cooking spray or additional butter for the pan
- Optional: Maple syrup or honey for serving

Instructions

1. Mix buckwheat flour, sugar (if you want to use it), baking powder, baking soda, and salt in a big bowl.
2. In another bowl, beat one egg and add buttermilk and melted butter. Mix until well combined.
3. Pour the wet mixture into the dry ingredients and stir until moistened; the batter should be slightly lumpy.
4. Preheat a nonstick skillet or griddle over medium heat; lightly grease with cooking spray or butter.
5. Pour about 1/4 cup of batter on a hot skillet for each pancake. When bubbles appear on top, flip and cook until golden brown on the other side.
6. If desired, serve them while they are hot with mixed berries and maple syrup or honey.

Nutrition (per serving):

Calories: 300 kcal Protein: 10g Fiber: 5g Iron: Good source

Green Smoothie Bowl

Preparation Time: 10 minutes Cooking Time: 0 minutes Servings: 2

Ingredients

- 2 cups of fresh spinach
- 1 ripe banana, sliced and frozen
- 1/2 avocado
- 1/2 cup of pineapple chunks
- 1/2 cup of almond milk
- 1 tbsp chia seeds
- Optional toppings: Sliced fruits (like kiwi or berries), granola, coconut flakes, nuts, or a drizzle of honey

Instructions

1. Blend spinach, banana (frozen), chia seeds, pineapple (crushed canned), almond milk and avocado in a blender. Blend until the puree becomes smooth. It should be mousse-like enough to eat with a spoon; change the amount of almond milk to make it as you like.
2. Divide the smoothie mixture into two bowls.
3. Top your smoothie bowls with sliced fruits, granola, coconut flakes, or nuts, according to your preference. Add some honey for taste if you need more sweetener.
4. Now, consume green smoothies immediately after they have been made while still cold.

Nutrition (per serving):

Calories: 300 kcal Protein: 8g Healthy Fats: High Calcium: 25% Fiber: 10g

Salmon and Quinoa Salad

Preparation Time: 20 minutes Cooking Time: 15 minutes Servings: 4

Ingredients

- 4 salmon fillets (about 6 ounces each)
- 1 cup of quinoa, rinsed
- 2 cups of water or low-sodium vegetable broth
- 2 cups of fresh spinach, chopped
- 1 medium cucumber, diced
- 1 red bell pepper, diced
- 1/4 cup of red onion, finely chopped
- 1/2 cup of cherry tomatoes, halved
- 1/4 cup of feta cheese, crumbled
- 1/4 cup of fresh dill, chopped
- 2 tbsp olive oil
- Juice of 1 lemon
- Salt and pepper, to taste

Dressing:

- 3 tbsp extra virgin olive oil
- 2 tbsp lemon juice
- 1 garlic clove, minced
- 1 tsp Dijon mustard
- Salt and pepper, to taste

Preparation

1. Bring 2 cups of water or broth to a boil in a medium saucepan. Add the grain, turn down the heat low, cover with a lid, and simmer for fifteen minutes until it absorbs all the liquid. Let it cool off for some moments.
2. In the meantime, season the salmon fillets with salt and pepper as you cook the quinoa. Heat olive oil over medium-high flame in a skillet. Place salmon into the skillet so its skin faces downward, and fry them on both sides for about five minutes each or until cooked through. Remove from the fire and allow it to rest for a while after cooling slightly so that you can easily flake it apart into large pieces.

3. Put cooked quinoa in a large bowl with spinach, cucumber, red bell pepper, red onion, cherry tomatoes, feta cheese, and dill.
4. Whisk together olive oil, lemon juice, minced garlic, Dijon mustard, salt, and pepper in a small bowl.
5. Pour dressing over salad and toss well. Finally, gently fold in the flaked salmon.
6. Divide salad into bowls or plates and immediately serve.

Nutrition (per serving):

Calories: 500 kcal Protein: 35 g Fat: 25 g Carbohydrates: 35 g Fiber: 5 g Calcium: 10% Vitamin D: 50% DV

<u>Turkey and Avocado Wrap</u>

Preparation Time: 15 minutes Cooking Time: 5 minutes Servings: 4

Ingredients

- 4 whole-grain tortillas
- 12 ounces cooked turkey breast, thinly sliced
- 2 ripe avocados, sliced
- 1 cup of baby spinach leaves
- 1/2 cup of shredded carrots
- 1/2 cup of cucumber, thinly sliced
- 1/4 cup of red onion, thinly sliced
- 1/2 cup of low-fat Greek yogurt
- 2 tbsp Dijon mustard
- 1 tbsp honey
- Salt and pepper, to taste

Preparation

1. Prepare a spread by mixing Greek yogurt, Dijon mustard, honey, salt, and pepper in a small bowl.
2. Put down the whole-grain tortillas on a plane surface. On each tortilla, spread with yogurt mustard mix.
3. Place turkey slices on each tortilla, together with avocado slices, spinach baby, carrot shredded cucumber slices, and red onion.
4. Wrap them tightly by rolling them up carefully to enclose the filling; you may use toothpicks if necessary.

5. Cut each wrap in half and serve right away, or wrap it with foil or plastic wrap for the go.

Nutrition (per serving):

Calories: 350 kcal Protein: 25 g Fat: 15 g Carbohydrates: 35 g Fiber: 7 g Calcium: 10%

Vegetarian Chickpea Stir-Fry

Preparation Time: 15 minutes Cooking Time: 10 minutes Servings: 4

Ingredients

- 2 cups of cooked chickpeas
- 2 tbsp olive oil
- 1 medium onion, chopped
- 2 cloves garlic, minced
- 1 red bell pepper, sliced
- 1 yellow bell pepper, sliced
- 1 cup of broccoli florets
- 1 cup of snap peas
- 1 carrot, thinly sliced
- 2 tbsp low-sodium soy sauce or tamari
- 1 tbsp sesame oil
- 1 tsp ginger, grated
- 1/4 tsp red pepper flakes (optional)
- Salt and pepper, to taste
- 2 tbsp sesame seeds
- 1/4 cup of chopped cilantro or parsley for garnish

Preparation

1. On medium heat, heat olive oil in a large skillet or wok. Sauté the onion with garlic until translucent.
2. Carrot, red bell pepper, yellow bell pepper, broccoli, and snap peas enter the skillet. Fry it for approximately 5 minutes or till vegetables become tender and crispy.
3. Then, stir well to combine cooked chickpeas with soy sauce, sesame oil, ginger, and red pepper flakes in a skillet. Keep going for another 2-3 minutes. Add salt and pepper as desired.
4. Sprinkle sesame seeds on top of the stir-fry immediately before serving alongside chopped cilantro or parsley.

5. For added fiber and nutrients, serve hot, either alone or over a plate of cooked brown rice or quinoa.

Nutrition (per serving):

Calories: 280 kcal Protein: 10 g Fat: 12 g Carbohydrates: 35 g Fiber: 9 g Calcium: 8% (DV)

Mediterranean Quinoa Bowl

Preparation Time: 15 minutes Cooking Time: 20 minutes Servings: 4

Ingredients

- 1 cup of quinoa, rinsed
- 2 cups of water or vegetable broth
- 1 cup of cherry tomatoes, halved
- 1 cucumber, diced
- 1/2 red onion, finely chopped
- 1 bell pepper, diced
- 1/4 cup of kalamata olives, sliced
- 1/4 cup of feta cheese, crumbled
- 1/4 cup of parsley, chopped
- 1/4 cup of extra virgin olive oil
- Juice of 1 lemon
- 2 tsp dried oregano
- Salt and pepper, to taste
- 1 avocado, sliced (for serving)
- 1/4 cup of hummus (for serving)

Preparation

1. Boil 2 cups of water or broth in a medium-sized pot. Enter the quinoa, lower the heat to low, cover it, and then simmer it for 15-20 minutes until all the liquid is absorbed. Stir with a fork and let it be cooled just slightly.
2. Mix cherry tomatoes, cucumber, red onion, bell pepper, and kalamata olives in a large bowl.
3. Mix olive oil, lemon juice, dried oregano salt, and pepper in a small bowl using a whisker.
4. Add cooked quinoa to vegetables. Drizzle dressing over top of salad; gently toss. Finally, mix in feta cheese as well as parsley carefully.

5. Serve the mixture in bowls; put avocado slices on top. Add some hummus to each dish, too.

Nutrition (per serving)

Calories: 400 kcal Protein: 10 g Fat: 20 g Carbohydrates: 45 g Fiber: 8 g Calcium: 10% (DV)

Chicken and Vegetable Skewers

Preparation Time: 30 minutes Cooking Time: 10 minutes Servings: 4

Ingredients

- 2 boneless, skinless chicken breasts cut into 1-inch cubes
- 1 zucchini, sliced into 1/2-inch rounds
- 1 yellow squash, sliced into 1/2-inch rounds
- 1 red bell pepper, cut into 1-inch pieces
- 1 green bell pepper, cut into 1-inch pieces
- 1 red onion, cut into wedges
- 8 wooden or metal skewers

For the Marinade:

- 1/4 cup of olive oil
- 2 tbsp lemon juice
- 2 garlic cloves, minced
- 1 tsp dried oregano
- 1 tsp dried thyme
- Salt and pepper, to taste

Preparation

1. Mix olive oil, lemon juice, minced garlic, oregano, thyme, salt, and pepper in a large bowl. Add chicken cubes to the marinade and toss them to coat the marinade evenly. Let it sit in the fridge for at least twenty minutes.
2. Heat your grill on medium-high.
3. Alternating between chicken and vegetables, thread marinated chicken, zucchini, yellow squash, bell peppers, and red onion onto skewers.
4. Grill for about 10 minutes, occasionally turning until the chicken is cooked and the vegetables have charred slightly.
5. Take off from the grill, after which they should be served hot.

Nutrition (per serving):

Calories: 250 kcal Protein: 25 g Fat: 10 g Carbohydrates: 15 g Fiber: 3 g Calcium: 5% (DV)

Spinach and Mushroom Quesadillas

Preparation Time: 15 minutes Cooking Time: 10 minutes Servings: 4

Ingredients

- 4 large whole-grain tortillas
- 2 cups of fresh spinach, chopped
- 1 cup of mushrooms, sliced
- 1/2 red onion, finely chopped
- 1 garlic clove, minced
- 1 cup of low-fat shredded cheese (such as mozzarella or cheddar)
- 1 tbsp olive oil
- Salt and pepper, to taste
- 1/2 tsp cumin (optional)
- 1/4 cup of salsa (for serving)
- 1/4 cup of Greek yogurt (for serving)

Preparation

1. Heat olive oil in a large frying pan over medium heat. Add the garlic and red onions, cooking until the onions become translucent. Also, add mushrooms and cook them till they get soft. Furthermore, add spinach and cook it until its wilting begins. Salt, pepper, and cumin are proper spices to season this.
2. Spread tortillas on flat surfaces. Sprinkle some cheese along half of each tortilla, then evenly distribute the spinach and mushroom mixture over that cheese. Then, fold over the other halves to make half-moon shapes.
3. Heat a clean frying pan/make sure your skillet is clean, then set aside/first, heat your skillet over medium heat/pull out a different/same(the) heating pan/frying pan with olive oil. Place one quesadilla in the skillet and cook for about 2-3 minutes per side until the tortilla becomes crispy and the cheese melts. Repeat with quesadillas left.
4. Divide each of these into wedges. Cut wedges from quesadilla. Serve with side salsa plus Greek yogurt adjacent to them.

Nutrition (per serving)

Calories: 300 kcal Protein: 15 g Fat: 12 g Carbohydrates: 35 g Fiber: 6 g Calcium: 20% (DV)

Shrimp and Broccoli Stir-Fry

Preparation Time: 15 minutes Cooking Time: 10 minutes Servings: 4

Ingredients

- 1 pound shrimp, peeled and deveined
- 4 cups of broccoli florets
- 2 tbsp olive oil
- 1 red bell pepper, sliced
- 2 cloves garlic, minced
- 1 tbsp ginger, grated

For the Sauce:

- 1/4 cup of low-sodium soy sauce or tamari
- 1 tbsp sesame oil
- 2 tbsp honey or maple syrup
- 1 tbsp cornstarch
- 1/4 cup of water
- 1 tsp red pepper flakes (optional)

Preparation

1. Whisk together soy sauce, sesame oil, honey, cornstarch, water, and red pepper flakes in a little bowl. Put aside
2. In a large skillet or wok over medium-high heat, 1 tbsp olive oil should be heated. Stir fry shrimp for about 2-3 minutes or until they turn pink and are well done; then remove them from the skillet.
3. The remaining olive oil is added to the same skillet with broccoli, red bell pepper, garlic, and ginger. Sauté this for approximately 5 minutes to ensure that vegetables are tender but crunchy.
4. Reintroduce shrimp into the pan onto vegetables after pouring sauce on top of it, then gently stir all that together. Let this cook further for some 2 more minutes as the sauce thickens.
5. Serve hot alone or in case with cooked brown rice or quinoa.

Nutrition (per serving)

Calories: 250 kcal Protein: 25 g Fat: 10 g Carbohydrates: 15 g Fiber: 3 g Calcium: 10% (DV)

Caprese Salad with Grilled Chicken

Preparation Time: 20 minutes Cooking Time: 10 minutes Servings: 4

Ingredients

- 4 boneless, skinless chicken breasts
- 2 tbsp olive oil
- Salt and pepper, to taste
- 4 large ripe tomatoes, sliced
- 8 ounces fresh mozzarella cheese, sliced
- 1/4 cup of fresh basil leaves
- Balsamic glaze (for drizzling)

For the Marinade:

- 1/4 cup of balsamic vinegar
- 2 tbsp olive oil
- 1 garlic clove, minced
- 1 tsp dried Italian herbs

Preparation

1. Whip balsamic vinegar, extra virgin olive oil, garlic cloves, and Italian seasoning in a large bowl. Put chicken in the mixture and refrigerate for a minimum of 15 minutes.
2. Set up a grill or grill pan and heat to medium-high. Take the chicken out of its sauce and salt it over before grilling. It is done in about 5 minutes per side batches until both sides are browned or the meat is cooked through. Let stand for a few moments, then cut into slices.
3. Arrange tomatoes layered alternatively with mozzarella cheese and basil leaves on a serving platter. Put sliced grilled chicken on top of or at the side of salad.
4. Just before serving, sprinkle olive oil on the salad along with some balsamic glaze.
5. Optionally serve this right away with crusty bread or even mixed greens.

Nutrition (per serving):

Calories: 350 kcal Protein: 30 g Fat: 20 g Carbohydrates: 10 g Fiber: 2 g Calcium: 20% (DV)

Egg and Veggie Wrap

Preparation Time: 15 minutes Cooking Time: 10 minutes Servings: 4

Ingredients

- 4 whole-grain tortillas
- 8 large eggs
- 1 tbsp olive oil
- 1 cup of spinach, chopped
- 1 red bell pepper, diced
- 1/2 cup of mushrooms, sliced
- 1/2 cup of cherry tomatoes, halved
- 1/4 cup of onion, chopped
- Salt and pepper, to taste
- 1/2 cup of shredded low-fat cheese (such as cheddar or mozzarella)
- 1/4 cup of salsa (optional for serving)

Preparation

1. Let olive oil get heated in a large skillet over medium heat. Put onions, mushrooms, and red bell pepper into the pan and sauté. Cook until tender, about 5 minutes. Add spinach and cherry tomatoes; cook until the spinach is wilted.
2. In a mixing bowl, beat the eggs, adding salt and pepper. Pour the vegetables and egg mixture into the skillet on low fire. Stirring occasionally, let them cook until set.
3. Warm tortillas using microwave or skillet. Spread an equal amount of egg-vegetable mixture on each tortilla. Sprinkle cheese over it.
4. Tuck in the sides of the tortilla, then roll from bottom to close, filling.
5. Cut wraps in two halves and serve with salsa, if desired, on the side.

Nutrition (per serving):

Calories: 300 kcal Protein: 18 g Fat: 15 g Carbohydrates: 25 g Fiber: 4 g Calcium: 15% (DV)

Chickpea and Vegetable Curry

Preparation Time: 15 minutes Cooking Time: 30 minutes Servings: 4

Ingredients

- 2 tbsp olive oil
- 1 large onion, diced
- 2 cloves garlic, minced
- 1 tbsp ginger, grated
- 1 tbsp curry powder
- 1 tsp ground cumin
- 1 tsp ground coriander
- 1/2 tsp turmeric
- 1/4 tsp cayenne pepper (optional, for heat)
- 1 can (14 oz) diced tomatoes
- 1 can (14 oz) chickpeas, drained and rinsed
- 1 cup of cauliflower florets
- 1 cup of carrots, sliced
- 1 bell pepper, chopped
- 1 cup of spinach leaves
- 1 can (14 oz) coconut milk
- Salt and pepper, to taste
- Fresh cilantro for garnish
- Cooked rice or naan bread for serving

Preparation

1. Over medium heat, heat olive oil in a big pot. The onion should be added and sautéed until transparent. Add garlic and ginger to the onion, and cook for another 1 minute.
2. Stir in curry powder, cumin, coriander seeds, turmeric, and cayenne pepper. Cook for about 60 seconds until it starts to smell fragrant.
3. Add the diced tomatoes together with the chickpeas. In addition, add cauliflower, carrots, and bell pepper to this mixture in the pot. Stir occasionally as it cooks for about 5 minutes.
4. Pour in coconut milk, then bring it to simmering point. Reduce heat and let it simmer for 20 minutes or till vegetables are tender.
5. Stir spinach leaves into the saucepan and cook till they wilt.
6. Salt and pepper can be used as flavorings on the curry according to taste preferences. Serve hot with some fresh cilantro garnish and cooked rice or naan bread.

Nutrition (per serving):

Calories: 350 kcal Protein: 10 g Fat: 20 g Carbohydrates: 35 g Fiber: 9 g Calcium: 10% (DV)

Avocado and Black Bean Salad

Preparation Time: 15 minutes Cooking Time: 0 minutes Servings: 4

Ingredients

- 2 ripe avocados, diced
- 1 can (15 oz) black beans, rinsed and drained
- 1 cup of corn kernels (fresh, canned, or thawed if frozen)
- 1 red bell pepper, diced
- 1/2 red onion, finely chopped
- 1/4 cup of fresh cilantro, chopped
- Juice of 2 limes
- 2 tbsp olive oil
- Salt and pepper, to taste
- 1 tsp ground cumin
- 1/2 tsp chili powder (optional)

Preparation

1. Diced avocados, black beans, corn, red onion, bell pepper, and cilantro should all be combined in a big bowl.
2. Lime juice, olive oil, salt, pepper, ground cumin, and chili powder (if used) should all be combined in a small bowl.
3. Drizzle the salad components with the dressing, tossing gently to moisten the avocado and beans without breaking them down.
4. To enable flavors to mingle, serve immediately or chill in the refrigerator for 30 minutes before serving.

Nutrition (per serving):

Calories: 300 kcal Protein: 8 g Fat: 15 g Carbohydrates: 35 g Fiber: 12 g Calcium: 5% (DV)

Grilled Salmon with Quinoa and Roasted Vegetables

Preparation Time: 20 minutes Cooking Time: 30 minutes Servings: 4

Ingredients

- 4 salmon fillets (about 6 ounces each)
- 1 cup of quinoa
- 2 cups of water or vegetable broth
- 2 zucchinis, sliced
- 2 bell peppers, cut into strips
- 1 red onion, sliced
- 2 tbsp olive oil
- Salt and pepper, to taste
- Lemon wedges for serving

For the Marinade:

- 2 tbsp olive oil
- Juice of 1 lemon
- 1 garlic clove, minced
- 1 tsp dried thyme
- Salt and pepper, to taste

Preparation

1. In a small bowl, combine the olive oil, lemon juice, minced garlic, thyme, salt, and pepper. After putting the salmon fillets on a plate and covering them with marinade, refrigerate for at least fifteen minutes.
2. Set the grill to medium-high heat and prepare your oven to 400°F (200°C).
3. Combine red onion, bell peppers, and zucchini with salt, pepper, and olive oil. Arrange them evenly on a baking sheet and bake for approximately 20 minutes or until they become soft and have a subtle brown hue.
4. Wash the quinoa in cool water. Boil two cups of water or broth in a kettle. Once the liquid has been absorbed, add the quinoa, lower the heat to low, cover, and simmer for 15 to 20 minutes. After turning off the heat, leave it for five minutes and fluff it with a fork.
5. Salmon fillets should be cooked to your preference after grilling for 5 minutes on each side.
6. Serve each salmon fillet with a portion of quinoa and a side of roasted vegetables. Garnish with lemon wedges.

Nutrition (per serving)

Calories: 500 kcal Protein: 35 g Fat: 25 g Carbohydrates: 35 g Fiber: 6 g Calcium: 5% (DV)

<u>Spinach and Lentil Salad with Feta Cheese</u>

Preparation Time: 15 minutes Cooking Time: 25 minutes Servings: 4

Ingredients

- 1 cup of dried green or brown lentils
- 4 cups of fresh spinach leaves
- 1/2 red onion, finely chopped
- 1 cup of cherry tomatoes, halved
- 1 cucumber, diced
- 1/2 cup of crumbled feta cheese
- 1/4 cup of olive oil
- 2 tbsp red wine vinegar
- 1 garlic clove, minced
- Salt and pepper, to taste
- 1 tsp dried oregano
- Lemon wedges for serving

Preparation

1. Once the lentils have been rinsed, please put them in a pot with two cups of water. Around 20 to 25 minutes of simmering or lowering the heat are required when the lentils are soft but not mushy. Empty and allow to cool.
2. Mix the cucumber, cherry tomatoes, red onion, and spinach in a big bowl.
3. Olive oil, red wine vinegar, minced garlic, salt, pepper, and oregano should all be combined in a small bowl.
4. Toss in the chilled lentils with the salad. Drizzle the salad with the dressing and toss to mix.
5. Add feta cheese to the salad and toss to combine.
6. Serve the salad in dishes and garnish with lemon wedges.

Nutrition (per serving):

Calories: 350 kcal Protein: 15 g Fat: 15 g Carbohydrates: 35 g Fiber: 15 g Calcium: ~15% (DV)

Quinoa Stuffed Bell Peppers

Preparation Time: 20 minutes Cooking Time: 40 minutes Servings: 4

Ingredients

- 4 large bell peppers (any color), tops cut off and seeds removed
- 1 cup of quinoa, rinsed
- 2 cups of vegetable broth or water
- 1 tbsp olive oil
- 1 small onion, diced
- 2 cloves garlic, minced
- 1 zucchini, diced
- 1 cup of mushrooms, chopped
- 1/2 cup of corn kernels (fresh, canned, or frozen)
- 1 can (15 oz) black beans, rinsed and drained
- 1 tsp ground cumin
- 1 tsp paprika
- Salt and pepper, to taste
- 1 cup of shredded low-fat cheese (cheddar or mozzarella)
- Fresh cilantro or parsley for garnish

Preparation

1. To make the dish, pour vegetable stock (or water) into a medium saucepan and bring it to a boil. Next, add quinoa, reduce the heat, and cook for 15-20 minutes until the liquid gets absorbed. Turn off the heat and fluff with a fork.
2. Preheat your oven to 375°F (190°C).
3. Then, you must heat olive oil in a skillet over medium heat. Fry onion and garlic till onion becomes transparent. Cook zucchini, mushrooms, and corn until they become soft. Add black beans, cumin, paprika, salt and pepper.
4. Blend cooked quinoa with the vegetables and bean mixture in the pan.
5. Pack peppers with this mixture (bell pepper filled with quinoa & vegetables). Put stuffed peppers on the baking dish.
6. After that, cover the baking dish with foil paper and bake it for about half an hour. Open up and sprinkle some cheese on each pepper; bake for ten minutes or until the cheese melts and the bell peppers turn tender.
7. Just before serving, garnish it with fresh cilantro or parsley.

Nutrition (per serving):

Calories: 350 kcal Protein: 15 g Fat: 10 g Carbohydrates: 50 g Fiber: 10 g Calcium: ~15% (DV)

Chicken and Vegetable Stir-Fry

Preparation Time: 15 minutes Cooking Time: 15 minutes Servings: 4

Ingredients

- 1 pound chicken breast, thinly sliced
- 2 tbsp olive oil
- 1 red bell pepper, sliced
- 1 green bell pepper, sliced
- 1 medium carrot, julienned
- 1 cup of broccoli florets
- 1/2 cup of snow peas
- 1 onion, sliced
- 2 cloves garlic, minced
- 1 tbsp ginger, grated
- For the Sauce:
- 1/4 cup of low-sodium soy sauce or tamari
- 2 tbsp oyster sauce (optional)
- 1 tbsp honey or maple syrup
- 1 tsp cornstarch
- 1/4 cup of water

Preparation

1. In a small bowl, combine soy sauce, oyster sauce, cornstarch, honey, and water. Set aside.
2. Heat 1 tbsp of olive oil in a large skillet or wok over medium-high heat. Introduce the chicken to the hot pan and cook until it turns brown and becomes ready for consumption. Remove the pan from the heat source and let its contents cool.
3. To this same skillet, add bell peppers, carrot, broccoli, snow peas, onions, garlic, and ginger, plus one more olive oil. Sautee vegetables till they become soft but still have some crispy texture.
4. Finally, put the cooked chicken together with its accompaniments like vegetables into the pot, mix it up with that sauce on top, and wait for it to thicken, taking 2-3 minutes more.
5. Serve warm as is alone or on top of cooked quinoa or brown rice.

Nutrition (per serving):

Calories: 300 kcal Protein: 27 g Fat: 10 g Carbohydrates: 20 g Fiber: 3 g Calcium: 5% (DV)

Greek Salad with Grilled Chicken

Preparation Time: 20 minutes Cooking Time: 10 minutes Servings: 4

Ingredients

- 4 boneless, skinless chicken breasts
- 1 tbsp olive oil
- Salt and pepper, to taste
- 1 tsp dried oregano

For the Salad:

- 4 cups of romaine lettuce, chopped
- 1 cucumber, diced
- 1 cup of cherry tomatoes, halved
- 1/2 red onion, thinly sliced
- 1/2 cup of kalamata olives, pitted
- 1/2 cup of feta cheese, crumbled

For the Dressing:

- 1/4 cup of extra virgin olive oil
- 2 tbsp red wine vinegar
- 1 garlic clove, minced
- 1 tsp Dijon mustard
- 1/2 tsp dried oregano
- Salt and pepper, to taste

Preparation

1. The chicken breasts are sprinkled with olive oil, salt, pepper, and dried oregano.
2. Before cooking, heat a grill or a grill pan over medium-high heat. Cook the chicken on each side for about 5 minutes until it is cooked. Let sit for a little while, then slice.
3. Mix lettuce, romaine, cucumber, cherry tomatoes, red onion, kalamata olives, and feta cheese in a bowl.
4. Combine olive oil, red wine vinegar, minced garlic cloves, Dijon mustard provence herbs, salt, and pepper in another small bowl.

5. Dress the salad with the dressing to combine. Additionally, add sliced grilled chicken to the salad.
6. One may optionally serve it along with pita bread and the salad straight away.

Nutrition (per serving)

Calories: 350 kcal Protein: 30 g Fat: 20 g Carbohydrates: 10 g Fiber: 3 g Calcium: ~15% (DV)

Whole Wheat Wrap with Turkey

Preparation Time: 15 minutes Cooking Time: 0 minutes Servings: 4

Ingredients

- 4 whole wheat tortillas
- 12 ounces thinly sliced cooked turkey breast
- 2 cups of mixed salad greens or baby spinach
- 1 tomato, sliced
- 1 cucumber, thinly sliced
- 1/4 red onion, thinly sliced
- 1/2 avocado, sliced
- 1/4 cup of low-fat mayonnaise or Greek yogurt
- 1 tbsp Dijon mustard
- Salt and pepper, to taste

Preparation

1. Ensure you have washed and sliced all your vegetables and are ready for cooking. If you are using Greek yogurt instead of mayonnaise, mix it with the Dijon mustard.
2. Put the whole wheat tortillas on a flat surface. Spread each tortilla with a layer of low-fat mayonnaise or the Greek yogurt and mustard mixture.
3. On every tortilla, lay even turkey slices. Put mixed greens on top and tomato slices, cucumber, red onion, and avocado.
4. Add in some salt and pepper to taste.
5. Roll up the tortillas tightly to encase the filling. When necessary, use a toothpick to hold them together.
6. Cut wraps in half and serve immediately, or wrap in foil or parchment paper for a convenient on-the-go option.

Nutrition (per serving):

Calories: 300 kcal Protein: 25 g Fat: 10 g Carbohydrates: 25 g Fiber: 5 g Calcium: 5% (DV)

Roasted Vegetable Quinoa Bowl

Preparation Time: 15 minutes Cooking Time: 30 minutes Servings: 4

Ingredients

- 1 cup of quinoa
- 2 cups of water or vegetable broth
- 1 small zucchini, diced
- 1 red bell pepper, diced
- 1 yellow bell pepper, diced
- 1 small red onion, chopped
- 1 cup of cherry tomatoes, halved
- 1 cup of broccoli florets
- 2 tbsp olive oil
- 1 tsp dried thyme
- Salt and pepper, to taste
- 1/4 cup of feta cheese, crumbled
- 1/4 cup of fresh parsley, chopped
- Lemon wedges for serving

Preparation

1. Under cold water, rinse the quinoa. Heat two cups of water or broth in a pot until it boils. Add the quinoa, cover, lower the heat, and simmer until the liquid is completely absorbed, 15 to 20 minutes. After removing it from the fire and letting it stand for five minutes, fluff it with a fork.
2. Start the oven at 400°F or 200°C.
3. On a sizable baking sheet, combine olive oil, thyme, salt, pepper, and broccoli with bell peppers, zucchini, red onions, and cherry tomatoes. When the vegetables are soft and faintly browned, roast them in the oven for 20 to 25 minutes after spreading them in a uniform layer.
4. Four bowls should be filled with the cooked quinoa. Sprinkle some of the roasted veggies over each.
5. Top each bowl with feta cheese crumbles and minced parsley.
6. Present the bowls beside lemon wedges for you to squeeze over the top.

Nutrition (per serving):

Calories: 350 kcal Protein: 12 g Fat: 12 g Carbohydrates: 50 g Fiber: 7 g Calcium: 10% (DV)

<u>Tofu and Vegetable Stir-Fry</u>

Preparation Time: 15 minutes Cooking Time: 15 minutes Servings: 4

Ingredients

- 14 oz firm tofu, pressed and cut into cubes
- 2 tbsp olive oil, divided
- 1 red bell pepper, sliced
- 1 green bell pepper, sliced
- 1 medium carrot, julienned
- 1 cup of broccoli florets
- 1 cup of snap peas
- 1 onion, sliced
- 2 cloves garlic, minced
- 1 tbsp ginger, grated

For the Sauce:

- 1/4 cup of low-sodium soy sauce or tamari
- 1 tbsp sesame oil
- 2 tbsp maple syrup or honey
- 1 tsp cornstarch
- 1/4 cup of water
- 1 tsp red pepper flakes (optional)

Preparation

1. If the tofu is not pre-pressed, put it into a clean kitchen towel or paper towel and put a heavy object on top to squeeze the additional water for about 30 minutes. Subsequently, cut the tofu into cubes.
2. Put one tbsp of olive oil in a big frying pan or wok over medium-high heat. Add the tofu cubes and cook until all sides are brownish and crisp. Please remove it from the skillet and set it aside.
3. Add one tbsp of olive oil in a frying pan again. Then add bell peppers, carrot, broccoli, snap peas, onion, garlic and ginger. Stir-fry for approximately five minutes or until vegetables have become tender yet crispy.
4. Mix soy sauce, sesame oil, maple syrup, cornstarch, water, and red pepper flakes in another small bowl.
5. Get the cooked tofu into the pan with vegetables. Dump the sauce on top of it and stir them up. Cook for another 2-3 minutes till thickened.
6. Serve hot, either as is or over a bed of cooked brown rice or quinoa.

Nutrition (per serving):

Calories: 250 kcal Protein: 12 g Fat: 12 g Carbohydrates: 25 g Fiber: 4 g Calcium: 20% (DV)

<u>Lentil Soup with Leafy Greens</u>

Preparation Time: 15 minutes Cooking Time: 45 minutes Servings: 4-6

Ingredients

- 1 cup of dried lentils (green or brown), rinsed
- 2 tbsp olive oil
- 1 large onion, diced
- 2 carrots, diced
- 2 celery stalks, diced
- 3 garlic cloves, minced
- 1 tsp ground cumin
- 1/2 tsp dried thyme
- 6 cups of vegetable broth
- 1 bay leaf
- Salt and pepper, to taste
- 2 cups of leafy greens (such as spinach, kale, or Swiss chard), chopped
- Lemon wedges for serving

Preparation

1. Heat olive oil using a large pot over medium heat. Put in onion, carrots and celery. Cook for about 5 minutes or until the vegetables are softened. Add garlic, cumin, and thyme; cook for another minute till fragrant.
2. Add the lentils which have been rinsed and drained into the pot. Pour vegetable broth and add bay leaf. Boil it and reduce it to a simmer; cover it on low heat for approximately 30-35 minutes or until the lentils are cooked through.
3. Stir in greens until they wilt, probably for about 5 minutes. Season with the desired amount of salt and pepper.
4. Take away bay leaf. Serve the hot soup with lemon juice squeezed into each bowl if necessary.

Nutrition (per serving, if serving 6):

Calories: 200 kcal Protein: 10 g Fat: 5 g Carbohydrates: 30 g Fiber: 10 g Calcium: 5% (DV)

Whole Grain Wrap with Hummus and Roasted Vegetables

Preparation Time: 20 minutes Cooking Time: 30 minutes Servings: 4

Ingredients

- 4 whole grain tortillas
- 1 cup of hummus
- 1 zucchini, sliced
- 1 bell pepper (any color), sliced
- 1 red onion, sliced
- 1 eggplant, sliced
- 2 tbsp olive oil
- Salt and pepper, to taste
- 1/2 tsp dried thyme or rosemary
- 1 cup of spinach or arugula leaves
- 1/4 cup of feta cheese, crumbled (optional)

Preparation

1. Preheat your oven to 400°F (200°C). Drizzle the zucchini, bell peppers, red onions, and eggplants with olive oil and sprinkle them with salt, pepper, thyme, or rosemary. Then gently place them on a baking sheet and let them roast for around thirty minutes or when tender and slightly browned.
2. The whole grain tortillas are then warmed in the oven for a few minutes or on a medium heat using a dry pan.
3. A nice layer of hummus is applied to every tortilla. The vegetables that have been roasted are added to the hummus. You can also include spinach or arugula to be sprinkled with cheese.
4. Wrap tightly, ensuring that the tortilla encloses the filling. One might consider cutting them in time halfway through to ease serving purposes.
5. Eat right away while still warm and fresh from cooking, or allow cooling before eating at room temperature.

Nutrition (per serving):

Calories: 350 kcal Protein: 12 g Fat: 15 g Carbohydrates: 45 g Fiber: 10 g Calcium: 10% (DV)

Salmon and Asparagus Foil Packets

Preparation Time: 10 minutes Cooking Time: 20 minutes Servings: 4

Ingredients

- 4 salmon fillets (about 6 ounces each)
- 1 bunch asparagus, trimmed
- 2 tbsp olive oil
- 2 cloves garlic, minced
- 1 lemon, thinly sliced
- Salt and pepper, to taste
- 1 tsp dried dill or fresh dill sprigs
- Lemon wedges for serving

Preparation

1. Preheat your oven to 400°F (200°C).
2. Cut four aluminum foil sheets, each about 12 inches long. Give every foil piece a little oil.
3. On each foil sheet, place a salmon fillet. Arrange the asparagus on one side of each package and place it next to the salmon. Pour some olive oil on the asparagus and fish. Season each with dill, salt, pepper, and minced garlic. Place slices of lemon over each fillet.
4. Pinch the foil's edges together to seal the packets thoroughly after folding it over the fish and asparagus.
5. After putting the foil packets on a baking sheet, bake them for about 20 minutes or until the asparagus is soft and the salmon is cooked.
6. Serve the salmon and asparagus with extra lemon wedges on the side after carefully opening the sachets and checking for steam.

Nutrition (per serving):

Calories: 300 kcal Protein: 35 g Fat: 15 g Carbohydrates: 5 g Fiber: 2 g Calcium: 5% (DV)

Quinoa-Stuffed Bell Peppers

Preparation Time: 20 minutes Cooking Time: 30 minutes Servings: 4

Ingredients

- 4 large bell peppers (any color), tops cut off and seeds removed
- 1 cup of quinoa, rinsed
- 2 cups of vegetable broth or water
- 1 tbsp olive oil
- 1 small onion, diced
- 2 cloves garlic, minced
- 1 zucchini, diced
- 1 cup of mushrooms, chopped
- 1/2 cup of corn kernels (fresh, canned, or frozen)
- 1 can (15 oz) black beans, rinsed and drained
- 1 tsp ground cumin
- 1 tsp paprika
- Salt and pepper, to taste
- 1 cup of shredded low-fat cheese (such as cheddar or mozzarella)
- Fresh cilantro or parsley for garnish

Preparation

1. Bring water or vegetable broth to a boil in a medium saucepan. Once the liquid has been absorbed, add the quinoa, lower the heat to low, cover, and simmer for 15 to 20 minutes. Take off the heat and use a fork to fluff.
2. Preheat your oven to 375°F (190°C).
3. In a skillet over medium heat, warm the olive oil. Sauté the onion and garlic together until the onion becomes transparent. Cook the corn, mushrooms, and zucchini until they are soft. Add the paprika, cumin, black beans, salt, and pepper and stir.
4. Add the cooked quinoa, beans, and vegetables to the skillet.
5. Place a filling of quinoa and veggie mixture inside each bell pepper. The filled peppers should be put in a roasting tray.
6. Bake for thirty minutes with the foil covering. Remove the cover, sprinkle cheese over each pepper, and return to the oven for 10 minutes or until the cheese has melted and the peppers are soft.
7. Before serving, garnish with fresh parsley or cilantro.

Nutrition (per serving):

Calories: 350 kcal Protein: 15 g Fat: 10 g Carbohydrates: 50 g Fiber: 10 g Calcium: 15% (DV)

Baked Chicken with Lemon and Rosemary

Preparation Time: 10 minutes Cooking Time: 40 minutes Servings: 4

Ingredients

- 4 boneless, skinless chicken breasts
- 2 tbsp olive oil
- 2 lemons, 1 juiced and 1 sliced
- 4 garlic cloves, minced
- 2 tbsp fresh rosemary leaves, chopped
- Salt and pepper, to taste
- Fresh rosemary sprigs for garnish

Preparation

1. Preheat your oven to 375°F (190°C).
2. In a big bowl, combine the olive oil, lemon juice, chopped rosemary, minced garlic, salt, and pepper. Toss to thoroughly coat the chicken breasts after adding them. Please give it a minimum of ten minutes to marinate.
3. The chicken breasts should be put on a baking dish. Lay down the lemon slices around and on top of the chicken. If desired, top with more rosemary leaves.
4. In a preheated oven, bake for 35 to 40 minutes or until the chicken is cooked and the internal temperature reaches 165°F (75°C).
5. Serve hot and garnish with fresh sprigs of rosemary.

Nutrition (per serving):

Calories: 250 kcal Protein: 27 g Fat: 12 g Carbohydrates: 3 g Fiber: 1 g Calcium: 2% (DV)

<u>Vegetarian Stir-Fry with Tofu</u>

Preparation Time: 20 minutes Cooking Time: 15 minutes Servings: 4

Ingredients

- 14 oz firm tofu, pressed and cut into cubes
- 2 tbsp sesame oil, divided
- 1 red bell pepper, sliced
- 1 green bell pepper, sliced
- 1 carrot, julienned
- 1 cup of broccoli florets
- 1 cup of snap peas
- 1 onion, sliced
- 2 cloves garlic, minced
- 1 tbsp ginger, grated

For the Sauce:

- 1/4 cup of low-sodium soy sauce or tamari
- 1 tbsp rice vinegar
- 2 tbsp maple syrup or honey
- 1 tsp cornstarch
- 1/4 cup of water
- 1 tsp red pepper flakes (optional)

Preparation

1. Cover tofu with a new kitchen towel or some paper towels. Put a weight on top to remove extra fluid for roughly 15 minutes. Then, cut the tofu into cubes.
2. Combine soy sauce, rice vinegar, maple syrup, cornstarch, water, and red pepper flakes in a small bowl.
3. Heat the large skillet or wok over medium-high heat by adding 1 tbsp sesame oil. Golden brown the tofu cubes on all sides, then transfer them from the skillet.
4. Put another tbsp of sesame oil into the skillet, then add bell peppers, carrot, broccoli, snap peas, onion, garlic, and ginger root. Stir-fry until vegetables are just tender and crisp, about 5 minutes.
5. Stir in the vegetables and mix the cooked tofu back into the skillet. Add sauce to be poured on top of it, and stir well together. Let it cook for an additional period of two to three minutes to allow its thickness to increase.
6. Serve hot, whether alone or over steamed brown rice or quinoa.

Nutrition (per serving):

Calories: 250 kcal Protein: 12 g Fat: 12 g Carbohydrates: 25 g Fiber: 4 g Calcium: 20% (DV)

Mushroom and Spinach Stuffed Chicken Breast

Preparation Time: 20 minutes Cooking Time: 30 minutes Servings: 4

Ingredients

- 4 boneless, skinless chicken breasts
- 2 tbsp olive oil, divided
- 2 cups of mushrooms, finely chopped
- 2 cups of fresh spinach, chopped
- 2 cloves garlic, minced
- 1/4 cup of low-fat cream cheese
- 1/4 cup of grated Parmesan cheese
- Salt and pepper, to taste
- 1 tsp dried thyme
- Toothpicks or kitchen twine for securing

Preparation

1. Preheat your oven to 375°F (190°C).
2. Take a skillet and pour in one tbsp of olive oil heated over medium heat; sauté mushrooms and garlic for tender mushrooms. Ensure it is done by adding spinach, which will wilt. After removing it from the heat, stir in cream cheese, followed by Parmesan cheese, before seasoning it with salt and pepper.
3. Butterfly the chicken breasts by slicing them horizontally, but not all through, so they open like a book. Flatten them slightly with a meat mallet.
4. Divide the mushroom and spinach filling among the chicken breasts, placing it on one-half of each opened chicken breast. Fold the other half over the filling and secure with toothpicks or kitchen twine.
5. Season the outside of the chicken breasts with salt, pepper, and dried thyme. Heat the remaining olive oil in a skillet and brown the chicken on both sides. Transfer to a baking dish.
6. Bake in a preheated oven for 20-25 minutes or until an internal temperature registers at 165°F or 75°C, which is checked using a thermometer to verify that it's well cooked.
7. Remove toothpicks or twine, allowing a few minutes to rest, then slice or serve whole after that.

Nutrition (per serving):

Calories: 300 kcal Protein: 30 g Fat: 15 g Carbohydrates: 5 g Fiber: 1 g Calcium: 10% (DV)

Lemon Garlic Shrimp and Zucchini Noodles

Preparation Time: 15 minutes Cooking Time: 10 minutes Servings: 4

Ingredients

- 1 pound large shrimp, peeled and deveined
- 4 medium zucchinis
- 2 tbsp olive oil
- 3 cloves garlic, minced
- Juice of 1 lemon
- Zest of 1 lemon
- 1/2 tsp red pepper flakes (optional)
- Salt and pepper, to taste
- 1/4 cup of fresh parsley, chopped
- Grated Parmesan cheese, for garnish (optional)

Preparation

1. Use a spiralizer to make noodles out of the zucchini. Set aside.
2. Heat 1 tbsp of olive oil in a big pan over medium-high heat. Add shrimp; season with salt and pepper; cook until pink and opaque, about 2-3 minutes per side. Remove shrimp from the skillet and put aside.
3. Into the same skillet, put minced garlic and remaining olive oil. Saute for one minute until fragrant.
4. Now, place the zucchini noodles into this skillet. Cook until they are barely tender, for around two minutes.
5. Put back the shrimp so they can go back together with the zucchini noodles in the skillet. Add lemon juice, lemon zest, and red pepper flakes (if you want), mixing well.
6. Remove it from the fire, sprinkle it with chopped parsley, and add grated Parmesan cheese (if you want). Serve immediately

Nutrition (per serving):

Calories: 200 kcal Protein: 25 g Fat: 8 g Carbohydrates: 8 g Fiber: 2 g Calcium: 10% (DV)

Spinach and Feta-stuffed Portobello Mushrooms

Preparation Time: 15 minutes Cooking Time: 20 minutes Servings: 4

Ingredients

- 4 large Portobello mushroom caps, stems, and gills removed
- 2 tbsp olive oil, divided
- 2 cups of fresh spinach, chopped
- 1/2 cup of feta cheese, crumbled
- 2 cloves garlic, minced
- 1/4 cup of red onion, finely chopped
- 1/2 tsp dried oregano
- Salt and pepper, to taste
- 1/4 cup of breadcrumbs (optional for added texture)
- 1/4 cup of grated Parmesan cheese (optional for topping)

Preparation

1. Preheat your oven to 375°F (190°C).
2. Rub one tbsp of olive oil on the top of Portobello caps and place them on a baking sheet.
3. Warm up the rest of the olive oil in a skillet at medium heat. Sauté garlic and red onion until they are clear. Add spinach to it until it is wilted. Season with oregano, salt and pepper. Turn off the heat and cool down slightly.
4. Combine feta cheese (and breadcrumbs if desired) with spinach mixture. Distribute this filling evenly into mushrooms' centers.
5. On each mushroom, scoop some grated Parmesan cheese. Place in a preheated oven for about twenty minutes or until the topping turn's gold while the mushrooms get tender.
6. Use these stuffed mushrooms as a main dish or a good side when served hot.

Nutrition (per serving)

Calories: 180 kcal Protein: 8 g Fat: 12 g Carbohydrates: 10 g Fiber: 3 g Calcium: 15% (DV)

Turkey and Vegetable Skewers

Preparation Time: 20 minutes Cooking Time: 10 minutes Servings: 4

Ingredients

- 1 pound turkey breast, cut into 1-inch cubes
- 2 zucchinis, sliced into 1/2-inch rounds
- 1 red bell pepper, cut into 1-inch pieces
- 1 yellow bell pepper, cut into 1-inch pieces
- 1 red onion, cut into wedges
- 8 wooden or metal skewers

For the Marinade:

- 1/4 cup of olive oil
- 2 tbsp lemon juice
- 2 garlic cloves, minced
- 1 tsp dried thyme
- 1 tsp dried oregano
- Salt and pepper, to taste

Preparation

1. Mix the olive oil, lemon juice, oregano, thyme, minced garlic, salt, and pepper in a large bowl. Toss to ensure even coating after adding the turkey cubes to the marinade. Allow it to marinade for at least half an hour (longer is better for maximum flavor).
2. Set your grill's temperature to medium-high.
3. Alternating between the marinated turkey and the veggies, thread the red onion, bell peppers, zucchini, and turkey onto the skewers.
4. After the turkey is cooked and the vegetables have taken on some char, place the skewers on the grill and cook for about ten minutes, flipping them over once.
5. Remove the skewers from the grill and serve hot.

Nutrition (per serving):

Calories: 250 kcal Protein: 27 g Fat: 10 g Carbohydrates: 10 g Fiber: 2 g Calcium: 3% (DV)

Eggplant and Tomato Bake

Preparation Time: 15 minutes Cooking Time: 45 minutes Servings: 4

Ingredients

- 2 medium eggplants, sliced into 1/2-inch rounds
- 3 large tomatoes, sliced
- 3 tbsp olive oil
- 4 garlic cloves, minced
- 1 tsp dried basil
- 1 tsp dried oregano
- Salt and pepper, to taste
- 1 cup of low-fat ricotta cheese
- 1/2 cup of grated Parmesan cheese
- 1/2 cup of fresh basil leaves for garnish

Preparation

1. Preheat your oven to 375°F (190°C).
2. Add salt and pepper to the eggplant slices after brushing them with olive oil on both sides. Place on a baking sheet in a single layer. Bake until soft and gently browned, about 20 minutes, flipping halfway through.
3. Sliced tomatoes, minced garlic, dried oregano, dried basil, and salt and pepper should all be combined in a bowl.
4. Arrange the tomato sauce, cooked eggplant pieces, and dollops of ricotta cheese in a baking dish. Continue layering until all components have been used, then finish with a layer of ricotta and tomatoes.
5. Add some grated Parmesan cheese on top.
6. Bake for 25 to 30 minutes in a preheated oven or until the dish is thoroughly baked and the top is golden brown.
7. Garnish with fresh basil leaves before serving.

Nutrition (per serving):

Calories: 300 kcal Protein: 12 g Fat: 18 g Carbohydrates: 20 g Fiber: 6 g Calcium: 20% (DV)

Chickpea and Spinach Curry

Preparation Time: 10 minutes Cooking Time: 20 minutes Servings: 4

Ingredients

- 2 tbsp olive oil
- 1 large onion, chopped
- 3 garlic cloves, minced
- 1 tbsp ginger, grated
- 1 tbsp curry powder
- 1 tsp ground cumin
- 1/2 tsp ground turmeric
- 1/4 tsp cayenne pepper (optional)
- 1 can (14 oz) diced tomatoes
- 2 cans (15 oz each) chickpeas, drained and rinsed
- 4 cups of fresh spinach leaves
- 1 can (14 oz) coconut milk
- Salt and pepper, to taste
- Fresh cilantro for garnish
- Cooked rice or naan bread for serving

Preparation

1. Heat the olive oil in a large pot over medium heat. Cook the onion until it becomes transparent and tender. Cook for a further minute after adding the ginger and garlic.
2. Stir in cayenne pepper, turmeric, cumin, and curry powder. Simmer for one minute or until aromatic.
3. To the pot, add the diced tomatoes and chickpeas. Simmer for a few minutes to let the flavors combine.
4. Add the coconut milk and spinach leaves and stir. Simmer until the curry slightly thickens and the spinach wilts, about 10 minutes. To taste, add salt and pepper for seasoning.
5. Add fresh cilantro as a garnish. Serve the curry hot with naan bread or cooked rice.

Nutrition (per serving):

Calories: 350 kcal Protein: 12 g Fat: 18 g Carbohydrates: 35 g Fiber: 10 g Calcium: 10% (DV)

Pesto Zoodles with Cherry Tomatoes

Preparation Time: 15 minutes Cooking Time: 5 minutes Servings: 4

Ingredients

- 4 medium zucchinis
- 1 cup of cherry tomatoes, halved
- 1/2 cup of pesto (homemade or store-bought)
- 2 tbsp olive oil
- 2 cloves garlic, minced
- Salt and pepper, to taste
- 1/4 cup of grated Parmesan cheese (optional)
- Fresh basil leaves for garnish

Preparation

1. Use a spiralizer to turn the zucchini into noodles. Set aside.
2. In a large skillet over medium heat, warm up the olive oil. Add the minced garlic and sauté until fragrant, about 1 minute.
3. To the skillet, add the zoodles. Sauté for 3–4 minutes or until they get somewhat tender.
4. Take the skillet off of the burner. Toss the zoodles in the pesto to ensure even coating.
5. Sprinkle with salt and pepper and stir in the cherry tomatoes.
6. Serve the pesto zoodles with fresh basil leaves and grated Parmesan cheese on top.

Nutrition (per serving)

Calories: 200 kcal Protein: 6 g Fat: 16 g Carbohydrates: 10 g Fiber: 3 g Calcium: 10% (DV)

Lentil and Vegetable Soup

Preparation Time: 15 minutes Cooking Time: 45 minutes Servings: 4-6

Ingredients

- 1 cup of dried lentils (green or brown), rinsed
- 2 tbsp olive oil
- 1 large onion, chopped
- 2 carrots, diced
- 2 celery stalks, diced
- 3 garlic cloves, minced
- 1 tsp ground cumin
- 1/2 tsp dried thyme
- 6 cups of vegetable broth
- 1 bay leaf
- Salt and pepper, to taste
- 2 cups of leafy greens (such as spinach, kale, or Swiss chard), chopped
- 1 can (14 oz) diced tomatoes
- Lemon wedges for serving

Preparation

1. Heat the olive oil in a large pot over medium heat. Add the celery, carrots, and onion. Simmer the veggies for 5 minutes or until they are tender. Add the thyme, cumin, and garlic and simmer for another minute.
2. Toss in the diced tomatoes, vegetable broth, bay leaf, and rinsed lentils. After bringing it to a boil, lower the heat to a simmer and cook the covered lentils for 30 to 35 minutes or until they become soft.
3. Add the leafy greens and simmer, stirring, for about 5 minutes or until they wilt. To taste, add salt and pepper for seasoning.
4. Take out the bay leaf. When serving, squeeze a lemon slice into each bowl.
5. Savor the soup hot, with crusty bread if preferred.

Nutrition (per serving):

Calories: 200 kcal Protein: 10 g Fat: 5 g Carbohydrates: 30 g Fiber: 10 g Calcium: 5% (DV)

Baked Salmon with Lemon and Dill

Preparation Time: 10 minutes Cooking Time: 15-20 minutes Servings: 4

Ingredients

- 4 salmon fillets (about 6 ounces each)
- 2 tbsp olive oil
- 1 lemon, thinly sliced
- 2 tbsp fresh dill, chopped (or 1 tbsp dried dill)
- Salt and pepper, to taste
- Lemon wedges for serving

Preparation

1. Preheat your oven to 375°F (190°C).
2. Put the salmon fillets in a baking dish. Season each fillet with salt and pepper after rubbing it with olive oil.
3. Arrange the lemon slices over the fish. Drizzle some chopped dill over the fillets.
4. When the salmon flakes easily with a fork, remove the baking dish from the oven and bake for another 15 to 20 minutes.
5. Extra lemon wedges should be served alongside the cooked fish.

Nutrition (per serving)

Calories: 300 kcal Protein: 23 g Fat: 20 g Carbohydrates: 3 g Fiber: 1 g Calcium: 2% (DV)

Grilled Chicken with Broccoli and Brown Rice

Preparation Time: 15 minutes Cooking Time: 30 minutes Servings: 4

Ingredients

- 4 boneless, skinless chicken breasts
- 2 tbsp olive oil
- Salt and pepper, to taste
- 1 tsp garlic powder
- 1 tsp paprika

For the Broccoli:

- 4 cups of broccoli florets
- 1 tbsp olive oil
- Salt and pepper, to taste

For the Brown Rice:

- 1 cup of brown rice
- 2 cups of water or chicken broth
- 1/2 tsp salt

Preparation

1. Combine brown rice, water, chicken broth, and salt using a medium saucepan. Bring to a boil, then boil the heat to low, cover, and simmer for about 30 minutes or until the rice is tender and the liquid gets absorbed.
2. Medium-high heat should be used to preheat your grill.
3. Chicken breasts should be brushed with olive oil and seasoned with garlic powder, pepper, salt, and paprika.
4. The chicken may be grilled for 6-7 minutes per side or until it reaches an internal temperature of 165°F (75°C). Remove from the grill and let rest for a few minutes.
5. Toss broccoli florets in olive oil, salt, and pepper. Grill alongside the chicken for approximately ten minutes, turning when necessary, till tender but slightly charred.
6. Then, slice the grilled chicken with broccoli and serve it with cooked brown rice.

Nutrition (per serving):

Calories: 400 kcal Protein: 35 g Fat: 15 g Carbohydrates: 30 g Fiber: 4 g Calcium: 5% (DV)

Stuffed Bell Peppers with Quinoa and Black Beans

Preparation Time: 20 minutes Cooking Time: 30 minutes Servings: 4

Ingredients

- 4 large bell peppers, any color, tops cut off and seeds removed
- 1 cup of quinoa, rinsed
- 2 cups of vegetable broth or water
- 1 can (15 oz) black beans, drained and rinsed
- 1 cup of corn kernels (fresh, canned, or thawed if frozen)
- 1/2 red onion, finely chopped
- 2 cloves garlic, minced
- 1 tsp ground cumin
- 1 tsp chili powder
- Salt and pepper, to taste
- 1 cup of shredded low-fat cheese
- Fresh cilantro for garnish
- 1/2 cup of salsa (optional for serving)

Preparation

1. Heat some water or veggie broth in a pot. Once the liquid has been absorbed and the quinoa is frothy, add it, lower the heat, cover it, and simmer it for 15 to 20 minutes.
2. Set oven temperature to 375°F, or 190°C.
3. Mix the quinoa with black beans, corn, red onion, garlic, cumin, chili powder, salt, and pepper in a big bowl. Add half the shredded cheese and stir.
4. Fill each bell pepper hollow with a spoonful of the quinoa and bean mixture. Arrange the filled peppers vertically in a baking dish.
5. Bake the peppers in the baking dish covered with foil for 25 to 30 minutes or until soft.
6. Once the cheese has melted and bubbled, uncover, top each pepper with the remaining cheese, and bake for five minutes.
7. Serve with salsa on the side, if desired, and garnish with fresh cilantro.

Nutrition (per serving):

Calories: 350 kcal Protein: 15 g Fat: 10 g Carbohydrates: 50 g Fiber: 10 g Calcium: 15% (DV)

Lentil Soup with Leafy Greens

Preparation Time: 15 minutes Cooking Time: 45 minutes Servings: 4-6

Ingredients

- 1 cup of dried green or brown lentils, rinsed
- 2 tbsp olive oil
- 1 large onion, chopped
- 2 carrots, diced
- 2 celery stalks, diced
- 3 garlic cloves, minced
- 1 tsp ground cumin
- 1/2 tsp dried thyme
- 6 cups of vegetable broth
- 1 bay leaf
- Salt and pepper, to taste
- 2 cups of leafy greens, chopped
- 1 can (14 oz) diced tomatoes
- Lemon wedges for serving

Preparation

1. Heat the olive oil in a large pot over medium heat. Add the celery, carrots, and onion. Simmer the veggies for 5 minutes or until they are tender. Cook for one more minute after adding the garlic, cumin, and thyme.
2. Toss in the diced tomatoes, vegetable broth, bay leaf, and rinsed lentils. After bringing it to a boil, lower the heat to a simmer and cook the covered lentils for 30 to 35 minutes or until they become soft.
3. Add the leafy greens and simmer, stirring, for about 5 minutes or until they wilt. To taste, add salt and pepper for seasoning.
4. Take out the bay leaf. When serving, squeeze a lemon slice into each bowl.
5. Savor the soup hot, with crusty bread if preferred.

Nutrition (per serving, if serving 6):

Calories: 200 kcal Protein: 10 g Fat: 5 g Carbohydrates: 30 g Fiber: 10 g Calcium: 5% (DV)

Quinoa Stuffed Acorn Squash

Preparation Time: 20 minutes Cooking Time: 45 minutes Servings: 4

Ingredients

- 2 acorn squashes, halved, and seeds removed
- 1 cup of quinoa, rinsed
- 2 cups of vegetable broth
- 1 tbsp olive oil, plus more for drizzling
- 1 small onion, finely chopped
- 2 cloves garlic, minced
- 1 tsp ground cumin
- 1/2 tsp ground cinnamon
- 1/4 cup of dried cranberries
- 1/4 cup of chopped walnuts (optional)
- 1/4 cup of crumbled feta cheese
- Salt and pepper, to taste
- Fresh parsley, chopped (for garnish)

Instructions

1. Preheat the oven to 400°F or 200°C. Place the cut side of the acorn squash halves on a baking sheet. Add olive oil, drizzle, and season with salt and pepper. Bake for 25 to 30 minutes or until the squash is soft.
2. Heat the vegetable broth in a medium saucepan until it begins to boil. After adding the quinoa, lower the heat, cover it, and simmer it for about 15 minutes until all the liquid has been absorbed. After five more minutes of cooking without a lid, fluff with a fork.
3. Warm up 1 tbsp of olive oil in a skillet over medium heat while the quinoa cooks. Add the onion and garlic, and cook for about 5 minutes or until tender. Cook for a further minute after adding the cinnamon and cumin.
4. After cooking, fold the cooked quinoa into the onion mixture in the skillet. Mix thoroughly after adding the walnuts and dried cranberries, if using. Season with salt and pepper.
5. Spoon the quinoa mixture into each side of the roasted squash. Add some crumbled feta cheese on top.
6. Re-bake the stuffed squashes for ten to fifteen minutes or until the cheese is melted and the filling is thoroughly cooked.
7. Before serving, sprinkle with chopped parsley.

Nutrition (per serving):

Calories: 325 Protein: 9g Fiber: 7g Calcium: 150mg Magnesium: 150mg

Spinach and Mushroom Omelette

Preparation Time: 10 minutes Cooking Time: 10 minutes Servings: 2

Ingredients

- 4 large eggs
- 1/4 cup of milk
- Salt and pepper, to taste
- 2 tbsp olive oil
- 1 cup of fresh spinach, washed and roughly chopped
- 1/2 cup of mushrooms, sliced
- 1/4 cup of grated cheese
- 1/4 tsp garlic powder (optional)
- Fresh herbs (such as chives or parsley) for garnish

Instructions

1. Beat the eggs with milk, salt, pepper, and garlic powder (if using) in a bowl until thoroughly mixed and slightly frothy.
2. Heat 1 tbsp of olive oil over medium heat in a nonstick skillet. Add them and sauté for three to four minutes when the mushrooms start to brown. Cook the spinach for one to two minutes or until it wilts. After taking the veggies out of the skillet, set them aside.
3. To the skillet, add the final tbsp of olive oil. Transfer half the egg mixture to the skillet and tilt it to ensure even distribution. Cook for two to three minutes or until the tops of the eggs are set but still somewhat runny.
4. One side of the omelet should have half the cheese sprinkled and half the spinach and mushroom mixture. Cook for an additional minute after folding the omelet in half over the filling. To make the second omelet, repeat with the remaining ingredients.
5. Place the omelet onto a platter and top with freshly chopped herbs. Serve right away.

Nutrition (per serving):

Calories: 290 Protein: 18g Fiber: 2g Calcium: 200mg Magnesium: 50mg

Turkey Meatballs with Zucchini Noodles

Preparation Time: 20 minutes Cooking Time: 30 minutes Servings: 4

Ingredients

For the Meatballs:

- 1 pound ground turkey
- 1/4 cup of breadcrumbs
- 1/4 cup of grated Parmesan cheese (rich in calcium)
- 1 large egg
- 2 cloves garlic, minced
- 1 tsp dried oregano
- Salt and pepper, to taste
- 1 tbsp olive oil for cooking

For the Zucchini Noodles (Zoodles):

- 4 medium zucchinis
- 1 tbsp olive oil
- Salt and pepper, to taste

For the Sauce:

- 1 can (14 ounces) crushed tomatoes
- 1 clove garlic, minced
- 1 tsp dried basil
- Salt and pepper, to taste

Instructions

1. Mix the ground turkey, breadcrumbs, egg, Parmesan cheese, oregano, garlic, salt, and pepper in a big bowl. Stir until thoroughly blended. Shape into meatballs about one inch in size.
2. Over medium heat, warm up the olive oil in a big skillet. Add the meatballs and cook for 10 to 12 minutes, flipping them over occasionally or until they are cooked and browned. Take out the meatballs and place them on a plate.
3. Add one more tsp of olive oil to the same skillet if necessary. For a minute, sauté the garlic. Add the basil and crushed tomatoes, then season with salt and pepper. Raise to a simmer. After adding the meatballs to the skillet, cook them for about 15 minutes while covered.

4. Spiralize the zucchini to make noodles while the sauce is simmering. Add zucchini noodles and olive oil to a large skillet heated to medium heat. Salt and pepper to taste, then sauté for 3–4 minutes or until the food is soft. Don't overcook.
5. Add the sauce and turkey meatballs after dividing the zucchini noodles among plates. If preferred, add more Parmesan cheese and fresh herbs as garnishes.

Nutrition (per serving):

Calories: 350 Protein: 27g Fiber: 4g Calcium: 150mg Magnesium: 50mg

Baked Sweet Potato with Chickpea Salad

Preparation Time: 15 minutes Cooking Time: 45 minutes Servings: 4

Ingredients

For the Baked Sweet Potatoes:

- 4 medium sweet potatoes, washed and pierced with a fork
- 1 tbsp olive oil
- Salt to taste

For the Chickpea Salad:

- 1 can (15 ounces) chickpeas, rinsed and drained
- 1 medium red bell pepper, diced
- 1 small red onion, finely chopped
- 1/4 cup of fresh parsley, chopped
- 1/4 cup of crumbled feta cheese
- 2 tbsp olive oil
- Juice of 1 lemon
- 1 tsp ground cumin
- Salt and pepper to taste

Instructions

1. Preheat oven to 400°F (200°C). Season the sweet potatoes with salt and olive oil. Put them on a baking sheet and bake for 45 minutes or until soft.
2. Chickpeas, feta cheese, red onion, bell pepper, and parsley should all be combined in a big bowl. Mix the olive oil, lemon juice, cumin, salt, and pepper in a small bowl. After adding the dressing to the chickpea mixture, toss to blend.

3. After the sweet potatoes are roasted and cooled slightly, carefully cut them open. Spoon plenty of the chickpea salad into each sweet potato.
4. If preferred, top the packed sweet potatoes with more feta cheese or parsley and serve right away.

Nutrition (per serving):

Calories: 380 Protein: 10g Fiber: 9g Calcium: 100mg Magnesium: 80mg

Green Goddess Juice

Preparation Time: 10 minutes Cooking Time: 0 minutes Servings: 2

Ingredients

- 2 cups of fresh spinach leaves
- 1 medium cucumber, chopped
- 2 green apples, cored and sliced
- 1/2 cup of fresh parsley leaves
- 1/4 cup of fresh mint leaves
- Juice of 1 lemon
- 1-inch piece of ginger, peeled
- 1/2 cup of water or coconut water (for added electrolytes)

Instructions

1. Thoroughly wash all the fruits, vegetables, and herbs under running water. Cut the cucumber into small pieces, peel ginger, remove apple cores, and slice them.
2. Pour the juice all together in a juicer containing spinach, cucumber, green apples, parsley, mint leaves (optional), lemon juice, and ginger. Add half a cup of coconut water or water to aid in blending. Process until everything is combined.
3. When it's done, the juice is stirred and mixed correctly. Serve at once in cups for the best taste and nutrient retention.

Nutrition (per serving):

Calories: 120 Protein: 2g Fiber: 5g Calcium: 60mg Magnesium: 30mg

Orange Dream Juice

Preparation Time: 10 minutes Cooking Time: 0 minutes Servings: 2

Ingredients

- 4 large oranges, peeled
- 2 carrots, peeled and chopped
- 1/2 inch piece of fresh ginger, peeled
- 1/2 tsp vanilla extract
- 1/2 cup of water or coconut water
- Ice cubes (optional for serving)

Instructions

1. Put the oranges, carrots, ginger, and vanilla extract in a juicer. Pour in the water or coconut water to make the blending process easier. Juice till it's smooth.
2. After juicing, thoroughly whisk the blend. Serve with ice cubes if you'd like a nice and refreshing drink.

Nutrition (per serving):

Calories: 160 Protein: 2g Fiber: 6g Calcium: 80mg Magnesium: 30mg

Berry Blast Juice

Preparation Time: 10 minutes Cooking Time: 0 minutes Servings: 2

Ingredients

- 1 cup of fresh strawberries, hulled
- 1 cup of fresh blueberries
- 1/2 cup of raspberries
- 1 small beet, peeled and chopped
- 1 apple, cored and sliced
- Juice of 1 lemon
- 1/2 cup of water or coconut water (for added hydration)

Instructions

1. The strawberries, blueberries, raspberries, beet, apple, and lemon juice should all be combined in a juicer. To make juicing more accessible, add water or coconut water. Juice till it's smooth.
2. Give the juice combination a good stir. To ensure optimal flavor and nutritional retention, serve right away.

Nutrition (per serving):

Calories: 150 Protein: 2g Fiber: 5g Calcium: 40mg Magnesium: 30mg

Tropical Delight Juice

Preparation Time: 10 minutes Cooking Time: 0 minutes Servings: 2

Ingredients

- 1 cup of fresh pineapple, chopped
- 1 medium mango, peeled and chopped
- 1 orange, peeled and segmented
- 1/2 banana
- 1/2 cup of coconut water
- Ice cubes (optional)
- 1 tsp lime juice
- Fresh mint leaves, for garnish

Preparation

1. Juice the orange, mango, and pineapple if you have a juicer. Another option is to use a blender. Smoothly blend the banana, orange, mango, and pineapple.
2. Add some coconut water to give the juice or blended concoction a tropical taste and extra moisture.
3. Serve the juice over ice or add ice cubes to the blender if you want it cooler.
4. Stir in the lime juice for a tangy flavor.
5. Transfer the juice into glasses, top with mint leaves that have just been picked, and serve right away.

Nutrition (per serving):

Calories: 150 kcal Protein: 2 g Fat: 0.5 g Carbohydrates: 35 g Fiber: 3 g

Beetroot Booster Juice

Preparation Time: 15 minutes Cooking Time: 0 minutes Servings: 2

Ingredients

- 2 medium beetroots, peeled and chopped
- 2 carrots, peeled and chopped
- 1 apple, cored and sliced
- 1-inch piece of fresh ginger, peeled
- 1 lemon, peeled
- 1/2 cup of orange juice (freshly squeezed if possible)
- Ice cubes (optional)

Preparation

1. Put the apple, ginger, carrots, beetroots, and lemon through a juicer.
2. Use a blender to puree all the ingredients until they are smooth if you don't have a juicer. You might need water or orange juice to achieve the desired consistency. Strain through cheesecloth or a fine-mesh screen to eliminate the pulp.
3. Mix in the orange juice to add more vitamin C and sweetness to the fresh juice.
4. To make the juice more refreshing, you might choose to serve it over ice.
5. Pour the juice right away.

Nutrition (per serving):

Calories: 120 kcal Protein: 2 g Fat: 0.5 g Carbohydrates: 28 g Fiber: 5 g

Green Calcium Boost Juice

Preparation Time: 10 minutes Cooking Time: 0 minutes Servings: 2

Ingredients

- 2 cups of kale leaves, stems removed
- 1 cup of spinach leaves
- 1 small cucumber, chopped
- 1 green apple, cored and sliced
- 1/2 cup of fresh parsley leaves
- 1/2 cup of broccoli florets
- 1 lime, peeled
- 1/2 inch piece of fresh ginger, peeled
- 1/2 cup of water or coconut water (optional for blending)

Preparation

1. Put the broccoli, lime, ginger, apple, parsley, cucumber, kale, and spinach in a juicer.
2. All the ingredients can be blended in a high-speed blender if you don't have a juicer. Add a small amount of water or coconut water to blend smoothly. Remove pulp by straining through cheesecloth or a fine mesh sieve if preferred.
3. The juice tastes finest when it's fresh. To get the most nutrients and flavor, serve it right away.
4. You can add a bit of agave syrup or honey if you'd like it sweeter.

Nutrition (per serving):

Calories: 80 kcal Protein: 3 g Fat: 1 g Carbohydrates: 17 g Fiber: 4 g

Tropical Bone Booster Juice

Preparation Time: 10 minutes Cooking Time: 0 minutes Servings: 2

Ingredients

- 1 cup of fresh pineapple, chopped
- 1 medium mango, peeled and chopped
- 1 orange, peeled and segmented
- 1/2 banana
- 1/2 cup of coconut water
- 2 tbsp ground flaxseed
- Ice cubes (optional)

Preparation

1. Juice the orange, mango, and pineapple using a juicer. Add the pineapple, mango, orange, and banana to a blender and process until smooth. This will give the mixture a thicker consistency, similar to a smoothie.
2. Add the coconut water to the juice or blended combination to give it a tropical taste and extra electrolytes.
3. Add the ground flaxseed to enhance the amount of omega-3 fatty acids that are good for bone health.
4. To make the juice more refreshing, you might choose to serve it over ice.
5. Drink immediately for the best taste and nutrient content.

Nutrition (per serving):

Calories: 180 kcal Protein: 2 g Fat: 2 g Carbohydrates: 40 g Fiber: 5 g

Almond-Broccoli Blend

Preparation Time: 10 minutes Cooking Time: 0 minutes Servings: 2

Ingredients

- 1 cup of broccoli florets
- 1 cup of unsweetened almond milk
- 1 banana
- 1/4 cup of raw almonds
- 1 tbsp chia seeds
- 1/2 apple, cored and sliced
- Honey or maple syrup to taste (optional)
- Ice cubes (optional)

Preparation

1. Blend broccoli florets, almond milk, banana, chia seeds, and apple in a blender. Process till smooth. To get the right consistency, thin out any excess mixture by adding almond milk.
2. If you want your drink sweeter, taste and add more honey or maple syrup.
3. You can pour the drink over ice or add ice cubes to the blender for a refreshing touch.
4. Drink the blend immediately to enjoy the maximum nutritional benefits.

Nutrition (per serving):

Calories: 250 kcal Protein: 8 g Fat: 12 g Carbohydrates: 30 g Fiber: 7 g

Citrus Kale Crush

Preparation Time: 10 minutes Cooking Time: 0 minutes Servings: 2

Ingredients

- 2 cups of fresh kale leaves, stems removed
- 1 orange, peeled and segmented
- 1 grapefruit, peeled and segmented
- 1/2 lemon, peeled
- 1 inch fresh ginger, peeled
- 1/2 cup of water or coconut water
- Ice cubes (optional)
- Honey or maple syrup to taste (optional)

Preparation

1. Put the kale, orange, grapefruit, lemon, ginger, and water or coconut water in a blender. Mix until smooth. Depending on your preferred consistency, you might need to change the amount of coconut water.
2. You can adjust the juice's sweetness to your preference by adding honey or maple syrup.
3. Add ice cubes to the blender or pour the beverage over ice in glasses to make the drink colder.
4. For optimal flavor and nutritional advantages, consume right away.

Nutrition (per serving):

Calories: 100 kcal Protein: 3 g Fat: 1 g Carbohydrates: 25 g Fiber: 5 g

Spinach-Banana Delight

Preparation Time: 10 minutes Cooking Time: 0 minutes Servings: 2

Ingredients

- 2 cups of fresh spinach leaves
- 2 ripe bananas
- 1 cup of unsweetened almond milk
- 1 tbsp chia seeds
- 1/2 cup of Greek yogurt
- Honey or maple syrup to taste
- Ice cubes

Preparation

1. Blend spinach, bananas, Greek yogurt, almond milk, and chia seeds in a blender. Process till smooth. Add a small amount of water to get the right consistency if necessary.
2. Add honey or maple syrup for a sweeter taste, then blend once more to combine.
3. Add ice cubes to your smoothie and blend until smooth if you prefer it cold.
4. After transferring the smoothie into glasses, serve it right away.

Nutrition (per serving):

Calories: 180 kcal Protein: 7 g Fat: 3 g Carbohydrates: 30 g Fiber: 5 g

Creamy Avocado Kale Smoothie

Preparation Time: 10 minutes Cooking Time: 0 minutes Servings: 2

Ingredients

- 2 cups of fresh kale leaves, stems removed
- 1 ripe avocado, pitted and scooped out
- 1 banana
- 1/2 cup of Greek yogurt
- 1 cup of almond milk, unsweetened
- 1 tbsp honey or maple syrup
- Ice cubes (optional)

Preparation

1. Combine the kale, almond milk, avocado, banana, and Greek yogurt in a blender.
2. Mix every item until it becomes creamy and smooth. You can thin out the smoothie by adding extra almond milk if it's too thick.
3. Taste again, and add honey or maple syrup if you'd like it sweeter.
4. Add ice cubes to your smoothie if you want it cold, then blend until the right consistency is reached.
5. For optimal flavor and nutrient retention, pour the smoothie into glasses and serve immediately.

Nutrition (per serving)

Calories: 250 kcal Protein: 8 g Fat: 15 g Carbohydrates: 25 g Fiber: 7 g

Blueberry Almond Zest Smoothie

Preparation Time: 10 minutes Cooking Time: 0 minutes Servings: 2

Ingredients

- 1 cup of blueberries
- 1 banana
- 1 cup of unsweetened almond milk
- 1/4 cup of raw almonds or 2 tbsp almond butter
- 1 tbsp chia seeds
- 1 tsp grated lemon zest
- Honey or maple syrup to taste (optional)
- Ice cubes (optional)

Preparation

1. Blend the banana, almond milk, chia seeds, lemon zest, almonds or almond butter, and blueberries using a blender.
2. Puree each ingredient in a blender until smooth. The smoothie will be naturally thick and cool if frozen blueberries are used. For a cold smoothie, you may use ice cubes if you are using fresh blueberries.
3. Blend again with additional honey or maple syrup added if required for sweetness.
4. To retain nutrients and maximize flavor, pour the smoothie into glasses and serve immediately.

Nutrition (per serving):

Calories: 250 kcal Protein: 7 g Fat: 12 g Carbohydrates: 30 g Fiber: 7 g

Spinach Mango Delight Smoothie

Preparation Time: 10 minutes Cooking Time: 0 minutes Servings: 2

Ingredients

- 2 cups of fresh spinach leaves
- 1 ripe mango, peeled and chopped
- 1 banana
- 1 cup of unsweetened almond milk
- 1 tbsp flaxseeds or chia seeds
- Ice cubes (optional)
- Honey or maple syrup to taste (optional)

Preparation

1. Blend the spinach, mango, banana, almond milk, chia, or flaxseeds.
2. Puree each ingredient in a blender until smooth. You can change how much almond milk you use to get your desired consistency.
3. Add honey or maple syrup and blend again if you want a sweeter flavor.
4. Add ice cubes to your smoothie and blend until the proper consistency is reached if you want it cold.
5. To experience the maximum flavor and nutritional advantages, pour the smoothie into glasses and drink immediately.

Nutrition (per serving):

Calories: 180 kcal Protein: 3 g Fat: 4 g Carbohydrates: 35 g Fiber: 5 g

Cranberry Beet Boost Juice

Preparation Time: 15 minutes Cooking Time: 0 minutes Servings: 2

Ingredients

- 1 medium beetroot, peeled and chopped
- 1 cup of cranberries (fresh or if using frozen, thaw first)
- 1 apple, cored and sliced
- 1 orange, peeled and segmented
- 1/2 inch piece of fresh ginger, peeled
- 1/2 lemon, juiced
- 1 cup of water or coconut water (for blending)
- Honey or maple syrup to taste (optional)
- Ice cubes (optional)

Preparation

1. Juice the orange, ginger, apple, cranberries, and beetroot if you have a juicer. Blend these ingredients until smooth, with water or coconut water if using a blender. If a more transparent juice is desired, strain through cheesecloth or a fine mesh screen.
2. For a zesty, new taste, stir in the lemon juice.
3. If you like your juice sweeter, add honey or maple syrup to taste.
4. Serve the juice over ice to enjoy it more refreshingly.
5. Consume immediately for the best flavor and maximum nutrient benefits.

Nutrition (per serving):

Calories: 120 kcal Protein: 2 g Fat: 0.5 g Carbohydrates: 30 g Fiber: 5 g

DAY	BREAKFAST	LUNCH	DINNER
01	Salmon and Avocado Toast	Chickpea and Vegetable Curry	Salmon and Asparagus Foil Packets
02	Almond and Chia Seed Pudding	Greek Salad with Grilled Chicken	Spinach and Mushroom Omelette
03	Almond and Banana Smoothie	Vegetarian Chickpea Stir-Fry	Lentil and Vegetable Soup
04	Green Smoothie Bowl	Chicken and Vegetable Skewers	Mushroom and Spinach Stuffed Chicken Breast
05	Greek Yogurt Parfait	Quinoa Stuffed Bell Peppers	Baked Salmon with Lemon and Dill
06	Tropical Paradise Protein Smoothie	Mediterranean Quinoa Bowl	Lentil Soup with Leafy Greens
07	Citrus Kale Crush	Caprese Salad with Grilled Chicken	Eggplant and Tomato Bake
08	Buckwheat Pancakes with Berries	Whole Wheat Wrap with Turkey	Baked Chicken with Lemon and Rosemary
09	Veggie Breakfast Burrito	Tofu and Vegetable Stir-Fry	Quinoa-Stuffed Bell Peppers
10	Avocado Toast with Smoked Salmon	Grilled Salmon with Quinoa and Roasted Vegetables	Spinach and Feta-stuffed Portobello Mushrooms
11	Coconut Yogurt with Tropical Fruit	Spinach and Mushroom Quesadillas	Turkey and Vegetable Skewers
12	Sweet Potato and Turkey Hash	Salmon and Quinoa Salad	Baked Sweet Potato with Chickpea Salad
13	Mushroom and Spinach Egg Scramble	Egg and Veggie Wrap	Grilled Chicken with Broccoli and Brown Rice
14	Quinoa Breakfast Bowl	Lentil Soup with Leafy Greens	Turkey Meatballs with Zucchini Noodles
15	Berry Blast Protein Smoothie	Whole Grain Wrap with Hummus and Roasted Vegetables	Stuffed Bell Peppers with Quinoa and Black Beans

16	Berry Chia Pudding	Roasted Vegetable Quinoa Bowl	Chickpea and Spinach Curry
17	Veggie and Feta Frittata	Avocado and Black Bean Salad	Lemon Garlic Shrimp and Zucchini Noodles
18	Whole Grain Cereal with Nuts and Berries	Spinach and Lentil Salad with Feta Cheese	Quinoa Stuffed Acorn Squash
19	Yogurt Parfait with Nuts and Berries	Shrimp and Broccoli Stir-Fry	Vegetarian Stir-Fry with Tofu
20	Spinach and Feta Omelette Roll	Turkey and Avocado Wrap	Pesto Zoodles with Cherry Tomatoes
21	Cherry Almond Overnight Oats	Chicken and Vegetable Stir-Fry	Chickpea and Spinach Curry
22	Spinach and Mushroom Omelette	Tofu and Vegetable Stir-Fry	Quinoa-Stuffed Bell Peppers
23	Cottage Cheese and Pineapple Bowl	Greek Salad with Grilled Chicken	Baked Salmon with Lemon and Dill
24	Blueberry Oatmeal Pancakes	Lentil Soup with Leafy Greens	Salmon and Asparagus Foil Packets
25	Overnight Oats with Almond Butter	Spinach and Mushroom Quesadillas	Turkey and Vegetable Skewers
26	Green Goddess Protein Smoothie	Chicken and Vegetable Stir-Fry	Lemon Garlic Shrimp and Zucchini Noodles
27	Almond-Broccoli Blend	Spinach and Lentil Salad with Feta Cheese	Quinoa-Stuffed Bell Peppers
28	Spinach-Banana Delight	Egg and Veggie Wrap	Baked Salmon with Lemon and Dill

www.ingramcontent.com/pod-product-compliance
Lightning Source LLC
Chambersburg PA
CBHW080725260726
48660CB00010B/3701